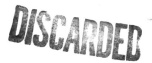
THE NAKED
TOOTH

THE NAKED TOOTH

*WHAT COSMETIC DENTISTS *DON'T* WANT YOU TO KNOW

COLLEEN OLITSKY, DMD

WITH

JASON OLITSKY, DMD

THE SMILE STYLISTS®

GREENLEAF
BOOK GROUP PRESS

This book is intended as a reference volume only, not as a medical manual. The information given here is designed to help you make informed decisions about your health. It is not intended as a substitute for any treatment that may have been prescribed by your doctor. If you suspect that you have a medical problem, you should seek competent medical help. You should not begin a new health regimen without first consulting a medical professional.

Published by Greenleaf Book Group Press
Austin, Texas
www.gbgpress.com

Copyright ©2011 Colleen Olitsky and Jason Olitsky

Distributed by Greenleaf Book Group LLC

For ordering information or special discounts for bulk purchases, please contact Greenleaf Book Group LLC at PO Box 91869, Austin, TX 78709, 512.891.6100.
Design and composition by Greenleaf Book Group LLC
Cover design by Greenleaf Book Group LLC and Base Art
Cover and interior photography © Jason Olitsky
Author photos © Tiger Studio
Six Months Smiles® photography © Dr. Michael Barr

Publisher's Cataloging-In-Publication Data
(Prepared by The Donohue Group, Inc.)
Olitsky, Colleen.
    The naked tooth : what cosmetic dentists don't want you to know / Colleen Olitsky, Jason Olitsky.—1st ed.
        p. : ill. ; cm.
    ISBN: 978-1-60832-057-8
        1. Dentistry—Aesthetic aspects. 2. Dental therapeutics—Planning. I. Olitsky, Jason. II. Title.
RK54 .O45 2011
617.69   2010935065

Part of the Tree Neutral® program, which offsets the number of trees consumed in the production and printing of this book by taking proactive steps, such as planting trees in direct proportion to the number of trees used: www.treeneutral.com

Printed in China

10 11 12 13 14 15 10 9 8 7 6 5 4 3 2 1

First Edition

Contents

*

Preface

I've written this book to serve as a guide for anyone considering improving his or her smile. It will educate you not only on the treatments available, but also on how to find a qualified dentist to perform the treatments for you. My hope is to decrease the number of smile makeover disappointments I see and hear about. Having your smile enhanced should be an amazing experience and my wish is that you find the right dentist the first time around.

I tell all of our new patient consults that I am there for them if they need anything or if they have any questions. Please feel free to contact me with any questions or concerns, I am more than happy to try to help.

Enjoy learning about what it takes to make your smile your strongest asset!

Colleen Olitsky, DMD, 904.273.1723
www.smilestylist.com, www.thenakedtooth.com

Introduction to a Better Smile

"I wish I had known!"

In more than nine years of practicing dentistry, I heard this sad lament over and over again from people who came to our smile makeover studio with cosmetic dentistry horror stories. As I tried to help patients recover from subpar dental work and read articles about badly made-over teeth in professional journals, I became increasingly appalled about the existence of so many dental nightmares.

I got so frustrated with this whole situation that I had to take action. I had to do something to help patients avoid poor cosmetic dentistry and get the smiles they truly want. I decided that the best way to educate patients was to write a book that would explain in simple language the procedures and pitfalls of cosmetic dentistry. *The Naked Tooth* tells it like it is. In this book, you'll learn about your options *based on the latest advances in cosmetic dentistry* and discover how to find a good smile artist.

You might well ask, "Why is this book necessary? Don't all dentists do good cosmetic work?"

The short answer is no, not all dentists can give you the smile of your dreams. In order to get the results you want, you have to do your homework and learn as much as possible about procedures and the cosmetic dental industry.

In the following chapters, I will teach you what cosmetic dentistry is all about. I will discuss the procedures—everything from porcelain veneers to laser gum lifts—as well as aesthetic considerations, including how to determine what you really want from your smile. I will also describe a process for choosing your cosmetic dentist and tell you how to maintain the smile you want.

Before you start your education, it is important that you understand why you need to take so much care to make sure you get the cosmetic dentistry you want.

A Disturbing Trend

From my experience and research, the cosmetic work being performed nationwide is simply unacceptable, and it seems to be getting worse. Ronald E. Goldstein, an author of cosmetic dentistry textbooks for dentists and founder of the American Academy of Esthetic Dentistry (not affiliated with the American Dental Association, or ADA), estimated that half of the $70.3 billion spent annually on dental work in the U.S. is related to cosmetic procedures. Of that, the Atlanta dentist said, redoing other dentists' inferior work and misdiagnoses accounted for $10 billion. As the number of cosmetic dental treatments increases, so does the number of victims of poor work.

Other academic dentists back these estimates. California cosmetic dentist Larry Addleson, past president of the American Academy of Cosmetic Dentistry (AACD), said that 15 to 20 percent of the patients in his San Diego practice are victims of poor work.

Gordon J. Christensen, a clinical professor at the University of Utah and owner of the for-profit, continuing-education Practical Clinical Courses in Provo, Utah, has frequently commented on the rise in incidence of botched work. He said the onus to arrest the rise of botched work falls on the ADA, which can recommend additional guidelines for cosmetic dentistry to state and local dental associations.[1]

However, the ADA, which represents the majority of the more than 155,000 U.S. dentists and advises the dental boards of each state, has stated that current ADA guidelines and state regulations provide adequate supervision for the safety of the public.

Getting Away with Shoddiness

This response from the ADA indicates how the majority of dentists trivialize the problem of bad or ugly cosmetic outcomes. To them, it only matters that the work is functional, meaning it meets a minimal standard of appearance. This reflects the ADA guidelines, which promote a standard of functional care but lack cosmetic standards.

In the meantime, dentists are getting away with shoddiness!

Now, I realize people have different opinions about what looks "good." It's possible the teeth makeovers I see and critique are exactly what the patients requested. That's fine. But I know

---

1 *The Wall Street Journal,* June 29, 2004.

how much better they can be, and most people don't—even other dentists. The bottom line is that these dental nightmares of botched cosmetics are totally preventable. And the best way to prevent dental nightmares is to educate yourself about cosmetic dentistry by reading this book.

Buyer Beware

What especially upsets me is that few people know that dentists can call themselves "cosmetic dentists" and claim they do smile makeovers without any training, experience, certification, or passion for doing them! Nor do patients know they need to do research before selecting the right dentist to perform a cosmetic treatment. Rather, they assume that when their general or family dentist tells them he or she can do cosmetics and recommends a certain treatment, that's the way to go. It's certainly easy to accept that without question or research—and millions do. Why? Because they trust their dentists. How would they ever know there's a wide range of talent and knowledge in cosmetic dentistry? Or they might believe they are "cheating" on their dentist if they seek cosmetics elsewhere. We've had clients come to us for smile makeovers, only to return to their dentist for regular care and be treated horribly for having had another dentist they had more confidence in perform the cosmetic work. What a hurdle for patients to overcome—all because their dentists won't refer out cosmetics.

Yet often these patients who have their cosmetic work performed by their general dentist end up unhappy with the results of their makeovers and wonder what to do next. Some live with it, bad-mouthing cosmetic dentistry to their family and friends; others seek dentists for a second opinion. Some end up paying twice—or never fixing their problem.

I urge you to do your complete research the *first time around* when considering a smile makeover. I see many "secondhand" patients who wish they hadn't rushed into the procedures they did and had asked more questions. Remember, years of practicing general dentistry is simply not the same as experience in smile makeover and enhancement dentistry!

I use the terms "smile makeover" and "smile enhancement" to mean two different things. A "smile makeover" is a full rework including eight or more veneers, perhaps in combination with procedures such as whitening, Invisalign, and gum lifts. I use the term "smile enhancement" to mean a smaller, less expensive procedure to improve certain aspects of one's smile. These include (and are not limited to) bonding and contouring, gum lifts, teeth straightening, whitening, or getting fewer than four veneers. Although these minor procedures aren't considered a full makeover, they can make a dramatic difference.

A Mark of Distinction: Smile Stylist®

My business partner and husband, Dr. Jason Olitsky, and I coined the term Smile Stylist® to refer to a dentist who has the passion and expertise for improving the quality of lives through smile makeovers. Our goal? To license the name Smile Stylist to those dentists who have continually advanced the art of smile makeovers—those who have embraced both the creative and the artistic aspects of this skill. We want Smile Stylist to become a household brand name, so when a prospective patient is searching for a dentist to perform his or her smile enhancement procedure, the patient will search for a Smile Stylist, not a "cosmetic dentist."

We think of our practice as a model Smile Stylist studio for helping people realize what's possible. My personal role is to welcome clients and provide a warm, comfortable environment for them. When they feel at ease, it creates an atmosphere in which both doctor and patient can develop a well-based, sincere relationship that gets better over time.

Part of this relationship hinges on the fact that Jason and I both interact with our clients before, during, and after treatment. Jason performs the cosmetic treatments because he's had more experience than I have. Yes, we have similar educations, but he showed a special gift and passion for smile makeovers years ago, and I've supported him in developing this specialty to a high level. As an aside, I wish other dentists who know they don't have either the education or the passion for smile makeovers would refer interested patients to a dentist who does.

This arrangement has served both us and our clients well. They frequently tell me how reassured they feel, having me available before, during, and after the procedure. I always tell them that Jason did my smile makeover. They like to see and talk to someone who's been through the veneering procedure and greatly benefited from it.

Total-Focus Environment

At our practice, the relationship starts with a consultation in which our clients are given a chance to articulate their long-term desires for their teeth. Then they receive the complete attention of both doctors during each procedure. We don't allow the typical interruptions of the dentist leaving the room while the patient is left waiting. Instead, having a total-focus environment ensures the best atmosphere for consistent results. It also shortens appointment times considerably and reduces the amount of anesthetic necessary for treatments. Our two sets of trained hands follow a rigorous protocol and thus minimize chances of potentially imperfect outcomes.

General dentistry practices that offer cosmetic, general, and family dentistry are confusing for the consumers. In our opinion, smile makeovers should be done with meticulous care by a highly trained expert in an environment exclusively dedicated to these specific treatments.

I hope that this book will give you the knowledge you need to get the smile you want and that you will support us in our efforts to raise the level of cosmetic dentistry in this country.

*

Chapter 1

The Importance of an Attractive Smile

Is your smile ready for life's runway? Is it a poor-quality smile that's hurting your career and your love life? You want your smile to do you justice whether or not you buy into the image-conscious, fashion-driven temptations of this world.

Chances are, you can easily tell when a person's smile doesn't match his or her face and personality—like a fashion mistake in the mouth. Many people are enhancing their smiles to complement their other great attributes. They understand that having bad teeth sends the wrong message to business and social partners. Fortunately, if you were not born with a "killer" smile, you can still have one, given you can fit a smile makeover into your budget.

You're Not Alone

According to the American Academy of Cosmetic Dentistry, 99.7 percent of Americans believe a smile is an important asset, and 96 percent believe an attractive smile makes you more appealing to the opposite sex. More important, 75 percent of adults believe an unattractive smile can hurt your chances for career success.

Psychologists say you communicate just as much with your mouth as you do with your body. Smiling is one form of body language that can make you more attractive. A number of studies show that a smile is generally perceived as more attractive than a frown; in other words, you're more approachable and desirable when you look happy. Two of the definitions of "smile" in *The Merriam-Webster Dictionary* are "to appear pleasant or agreeable" and "to bestow approval"—both important attributes in your personal life as well as the business world.

A recent study (by Harris Interactive, the global leader in online market research) of a representative sample of 1,000 American adults, both women and men ages between 18 and 50 years of age, found the following:

- Teeth are the number one facial feature people would change if they were to change something.
- Seventy-one percent of those polled believe people with a nice smile make friends more easily.
- Eighty-four percent think an attractive smile is important for meeting Mister or Miss Right.
- Ninety-four percent said they're likely to notice a person's smile when they meet the person for the first time, whereas people are less likely to notice someone's height, eyes, or figure.

- Eighty-five percent consider a person's smile to be *very important* when meeting someone for the first time.
- More than one-third agree that bad teeth overshadow the rest of a person's appearance.
- Sixty-four percent agree that people with a nice smile are more outgoing.
- Seventy-seven percent think that having discolored teeth as an adult makes a person feel self-conscious.
- Eighty-seven percent think a person's smile is very important to their self-esteem.
- More than one-third would not likely set up their best friend on a blind date with someone who has bad teeth.
- One-third would not be likely to kiss someone with bad teeth.
- Eighty-six percent think people with good teeth are more attractive than people with bad teeth.

Haven't you been influenced by the simple art of smiling at one time or another? Maybe you were approached by a person of the opposite sex who asked for a date or invited you for a cup of coffee. If so, weren't your chances of accepting the invitation greater if the person gave you a friendly smile?

An old Chinese proverb says that the person who cannot smile should not set up a shop. In business, that smile is a signal of welcome to potential patrons, showing them they're appreciated and respected.

Businesspeople from all walks of life have discovered the importance of a smile. Why? A smile attracts customers because it not only breaks down the barriers between people but also projects the salesman's confidence in himself and his products.

A Humorous Nature Requires Smiling

Numerous surveys have found that having a humorous nature is one of the top five qualities of men that attracts others. Yet it can be difficult for a man to attract many friends if he's unable to smile. More and more, the power of a smile is being extolled to businesspeople around the country and the world. As competition heats up, service and friendliness—in addition to price—factor into "winning" the client. That old saying "People do business with people they like" is infinitely true.

Dale Carnegie, a pioneer in self-development, devoted an entire section in his book *How to Win Friends and Influence People* to the importance of having a nice smile. There, he listed smiling as one of the six principles in getting people to like you, and described a smile as something "so valuable, it can't be bought." Maybe not, but a smile certainly can be improved.

Beauty = Goodness

Bombarded by images of beautiful people in movies, on television, and in magazines, society has become convinced and conditioned to believe that "beauty equals being good." This powerful message is ancient. Greek philosophers explained it first, and hundreds of recent studies prove that this idea affects our lives in untold ways. Attractive people are judged to be smarter, friendlier, more honest and trustworthy, more successful and happy, and in possession of just about every other "good" trait. Our world is so competitive today—both socially and sexually—that looking our best has become a necessity.

An independent U.S. study conducted on behalf of the AACD in 2004 discovered the following:

- Nearly one hundred percent believe a smile is an important social asset.

- Ninety-six percent of adults believe an attractive smile makes a person more appealing to members of the opposite sex.

- Seventy-four percent of adults feel an unattractive smile can hurt a person's chances for career success.

When asked, "What is the first thing you notice in a person's smile?" common responses were:

- Straightness
- Whiteness and color of teeth
- Cleanliness of teeth
- Sincerity of smile
- Any missing teeth
- Sparkle of smile

When asked, "What types of things make you consider a smile unattractive?" common responses were:

- Discolored, yellow, or stained teeth
- Missing teeth
- Crooked teeth
- Decaying teeth and cavities
- Gaps and spaces in teeth
- Dirty teeth

And, finally, when respondents were asked, "What would you most like to improve about your smile?" the most common response was:

- Whiter, brighter teeth

So what happens when your teeth are yellow and you become too self-conscious even to smile? Not only are you unhappy, but your ability to succeed becomes impaired. That smile concerns you and your confidence as a person while also affecting your ability to earn a living.

Whether your goal is being attractive, improving your career, or just feeling better about yourself, a new smile can make a dramatic difference in your life. Our clients tell me their increased confidence from a new smile has been a catalyst for many life-altering changes in career advancement, health and fitness, and continuing to improve their lives.

Are You Happy with Your Smile?

A smile is a person's most important facial expression, an important part of a first impression, and something often remembered long after you've left the room. However, some people try *not* to smile or they feel self-conscious when they do, largely because of imperfections with their teeth. If this describes you, you no longer have to settle for stained, chipped, missing, or misshapen teeth. Advances in dentistry have solved these problems; you now have choices that will help you smile with confidence.

If you're unhappy with your smile or you feel self-conscious when you laugh or meet people, then do something about it. Most of my clients declare that their only regret after their cosmetic treatments is they didn't do it sooner. Looks do count in today's society, and fair or not, you're judged by your smile and how you do or don't use that smile. Even if you say you don't care what you look like, other people do. Admittedly, dwelling on what your teeth look like can be considered superficial, but so can focusing on your haircut, clothes, car, and house.

The following chapters of this book present the different types of cosmetic dental treatments available and the spectacular results that can be achieved. These treatments may be used by themselves or in combination to achieve a gorgeous smile. It's up to you to discuss your goals and budget with the dentists you interview so you can choose what's right for you. Some people need only minor tweaking; others need an entire mouth makeover. A dentist with training and experience in smile enhancement will help you sort out your options.

But first, check out a few examples of how a new smile helped our clients achieve the confidence they always knew they had inside themselves. It's amazing to witness not only the physical transformation but the emotional one, too. Although they were happy people, they weren't able to show it because they felt self-conscious about their smiles. Some clients said they avoided social situations so they wouldn't have to be embarrassed. Others told us they wanted to be able to show their families and friends how truly happy they were on the inside.

What a gift we are privileged to give!

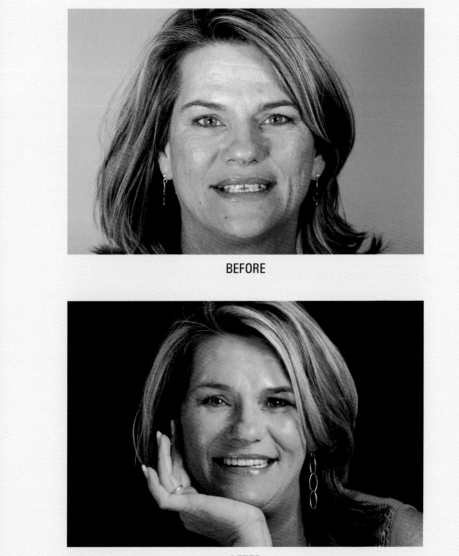

BEFORE

AFTER

Tina actually wrote $40,000 into her business plan to fix her teeth when starting a jewelry business. That gave her a nice smile to reflect how successful she knew she could be.

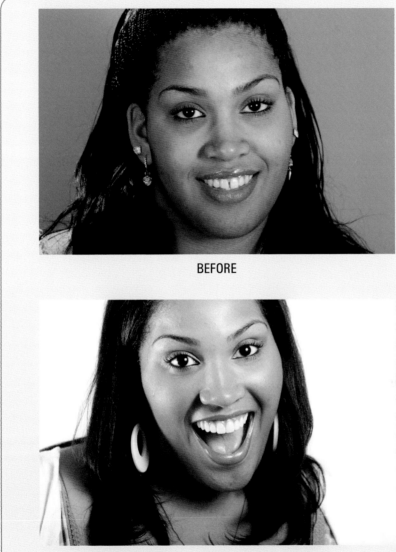

BEFORE

AFTER

Colby received 10 veneers on her top teeth and 10 on the bottom to give her the confidence she needed to fully participate at college with her friends and at home with her family.

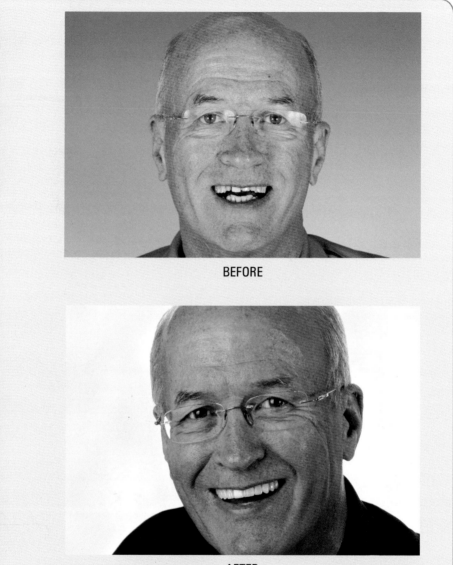

BEFORE

AFTER

Bill received a whole smile makeover and has enjoyed using his smile, in both his business and his social life.

✳

Chapter 2

A New Smile with Porcelain Veneers

Our Smile Stylist studio is best known for its porcelain veneers, so this chapter is based on our own experiences as well as feedback from our clients. It will give you a good idea of the issues and techniques involved with veneers.

Veneers are ultra-thin, custom-made porcelain pieces that are permanently bonded to the teeth. They've become increasingly popular and provide a durable option for changing the size, shape, position, and color of teeth. Veneers are used to close gaps, straighten teeth, replace worn edges, or resurface discolored teeth. The best candidates for veneers are people whose teeth are healthy and free from periodontal disease. However, cavities can often be repaired at the time of veneer preparation.

A veneer covers mainly the visible front part of the tooth and wraps slightly over the biting edge. There's no black-and-white distinction between crowns and veneers. Sometimes a veneer will wrap over to the tongue side of a tooth to help the bite, and sometimes a veneer will wrap around the entire tooth like a crown. It doesn't matter whether it's called a "crown" or a "veneer" because, to the observer, these will look identical. For example, I was born without my laterals, the two teeth next to the front ones. My new smile consists of bridges, crowns, and veneers, but I defy anyone to tell the difference. You do want to ensure, however, that your dentist uses the most conservative techniques possible.

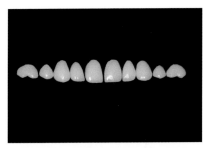

✻ These are 10 veneers, which are thin pieces of porcelain used to transform smiles.

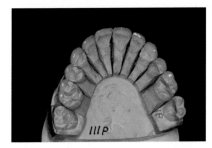

✻ This photo shows how the veneers wrap over the edges of the teeth.

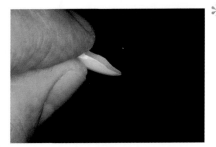

✻ This shows the thinness of the porcelain veneer.

As much art goes into enhancing a smile as technical skill and knowledge, so choose an expert dentist who focuses on artistically creating natural-looking and natural-feeling veneers. Dentists can address the tiniest details that make the difference between fake-looking teeth and a naturally beautiful smile with added flare. Our best contribution to date is the ability to create the market-driven whiter smiles using veneers that maintain a natural appearance.

The Story of RENA (Replicate and Enhance Natural Aesthetics)

In speaking with many clients, I've found they want their teeth to be white, yet natural, which is why we developed RENA. We design a person's smile so it looks like he or she was born with it. We tell our clients the goal is to have people think, "Wow! Isn't that person lucky to be blessed with such a gorgeous smile?" Sure, they'll probably think they had braces when they were young and they'll suspect they bleach their teeth to whiten them—but they'll believe they were born with that smile. And every single patient exclaims, "Yes, that's what I want!"

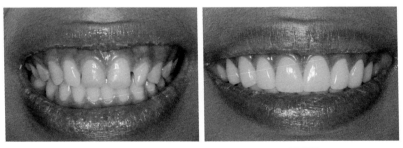

BEFORE   **AFTER**

Advanced techniques allow dentists to mimic and enhance nature, making veneers look like teeth, not veneers. Many of our clients were afraid to get veneers because they knew someone who had them and could immediately tell that the person had cosmetic dentistry treatments.

When we at Smile Stylist perform a smile design, our clients' friends and family think they look different, better, or younger, but either they can't tell why or they think they just got their teeth straightened or whitened. Because the smile looks so natural, it never occurs to others that the teeth are veneers.

How is this accomplished? It's because of a technique to measure the lengths, sizes, and proportions of people's natural teeth. We are able to evaluate what the smile would look like if the teeth had come in perfectly and in the most aesthetic places. We then decide on aspects of "flare" that add character to the smile based on our knowledge and the person's personality and desires. Examples include the shade of whiteness and the shapes of the teeth, which can be flirty and fun, sexy and exotic, masculine or feminine.

We are able to assess the person's facial characteristics, including the angles of the face and shapes of the eyes, and we then highlight these natural characteristics. For example, some clients want to make their smiles more fun, youthful, and flirtatious, while others want a more sexy, exotic smile. Most men prefer a more masculine smile than they have. Working with one of the most talented ceramists in the world to create our veneers out of the strongest materials makes a difference. The result? You look as though you were born with a beautiful smile!

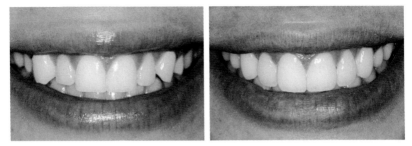

BEFORE   AFTER

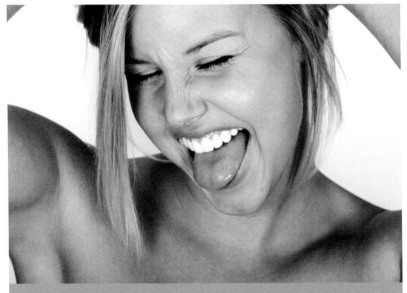

Lyndsay wanted a more elegant, flirtatious, feminine smile. These characteristics are highlighted with rounded, oval-shaped, soft teeth and a happy, fresh look.

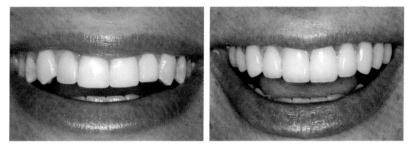

BEFORE   AFTER

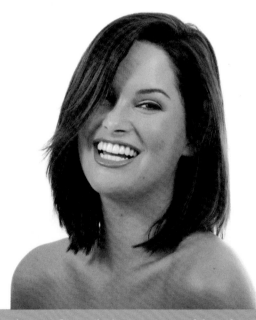

Whitney, winner of *America's Next Top Model* Cycle 10, wanted a more exotic, sexy look. We replaced her old bonding and covered her scars from orthodontics with 10 veneers to achieve her goals. The result? Natural, not commercial-looking.

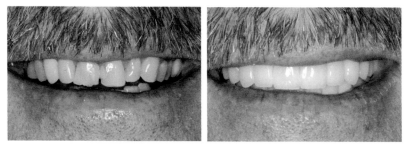

BEFORE   **AFTER**

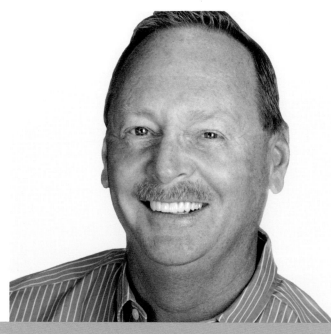

Bill wanted to have a more masculine smile, which is achieved with more angular, even, and squared-off teeth. This helped him feel more confident smiling with his family, friends, and colleagues.

The Three Most Common Concerns and Myths

What I hear most often from smile makeover clients are the following comments:

- "I don't want my teeth ground down."
- "I don't want them to look big, bulky, or fake."
- "My dentist told me veneers don't work."

Let's address each of these concerns.

Concern or Myth #1: "I don't want my teeth ground down."

Too often, we hear during consultations that patients don't want veneers because they don't want their teeth ground down. Perhaps a friend had some kind of aggressive work done to his teeth and the dentist ground his teeth down to "little pegs." So instead of having the smile they dream of, these people deal with what they have and never really like their teeth.

The truth is, veneer preparations are not as aggressive as typical crown preps. I show clients many different photos of what teeth look like when they're reshaped—minimally in most cases. Here's the real problem: Many dentists still grind down the teeth to pegs because they have no training in veneers. What a crime!

But let's get something straight: Dentists have been grinding down healthy tooth structure since the beginning of the profession. In dental school, we are taught to do bridges by aggressively grinding down two healthy teeth in order to replace a missing one. Dentists also extract healthy teeth in both children and adults for cosmetic purposes when putting on braces. That's the whole tooth, not just 0.5 mm of enamel that may be discolored or ugly anyway.

Examples

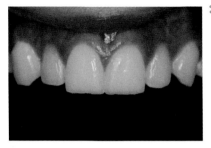

✳ This photo shows a close-up before the makeover.

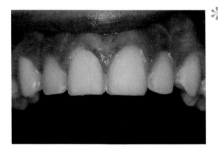

✳ This photo shows the preparation of the teeth and how much tooth structure may be removed before placing the veneers. Obviously, the teeth are not ground down to pegs or spikes.

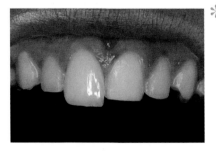

✳ This photo shows the application of one veneer and indicates how it melts away at the gum line—no bulkiness or discoloration.

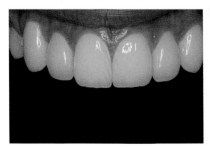

✳ This photo shows a close-up of the final veneers cemented in. Notice how natural they look.

No-prep or Prepless Veneers

Typically, removing some tooth structure in order to apply a crown or filling or veneer is needed to place and retain the restoration. Conservation is key with cosmetic dentistry, and in recent years new developments in techniques and materials have resulted in a new way to look at no-prep veneers. This concept initially drew negative concerns about the veneers being too bulky or overly contoured; however, when using a talented dentist and ceramist, the results can be stunning! Dentists agree that case selection—knowing when this technique will work and when it will not—is most important here.

There are a number of people who may be good candidates for no-prep veneers. People with small teeth can benefit from this additive approach to create aesthetically pleasing and natural-looking restorations without having any tooth structure removed. People have small teeth for a number of reasons. These range from genetics to tooth wear to spacing to acid erosion, to name a few. People with narrow smiles are also good candidates because we want to widen or bring out the smile.

Not every smile can be enhanced with no-prep veneers. Certain situations cannot be corrected, such as teeth that are too big, teeth that are positioned forward, and teeth that are out of alignment or in improper positions. If orthodontic treatment is refused, then some tooth structure must be removed to help correct or camouflage these flaws; otherwise, these illusions will come with some limitations. An ideal result may not be possible.

Only an experienced, trained dentist can help you decide which treatment option is best for you: traditional veneers, no-prep veneers, or even a combo of traditional and no-prep veneers. Your dentist will be able to choose the most conservative option while still obtaining the most beautiful and natural-looking smile possible.

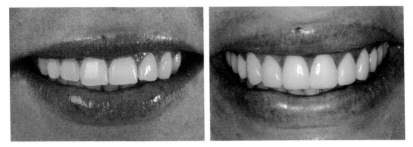

BEFORE   AFTER

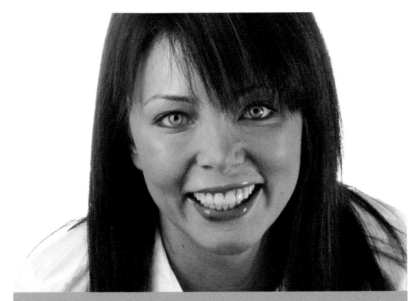

Alex, who models in Florida and Texas, wanted a conservative option to whiten her teeth and correct the chips and wear that began to prematurely age her smile. We used no-prep veneers to achieve her goals and enhance her smile.

Concern or Myth #2: "I don't want them to look big, bulky, or fake."

People are moving away from the bright white "Hollywood" look; they want beautiful, natural-looking smiles. Nobody, even dentists, have been able to detect that the veneers I have on my teeth are porcelain because, today, it's possible for a dentist and the lab to do a fantastic job with color and vitality. They strive to make porcelain look natural, regardless of the color.

This is why it's important to examine many photos before selecting a dentist. If the dentist's photos show big, bulky veneers, then don't go there, because that's what you'll get. I've read about some dentists who actually make their veneers crooked so they look more natural. That's ridiculous! People spend millions on braces because they want *straight* teeth. These dentists just create unnatural-looking veneers, so the only way to make them look more natural is to make them crooked. I don't know about you, but I wouldn't want to pay for crooked teeth!

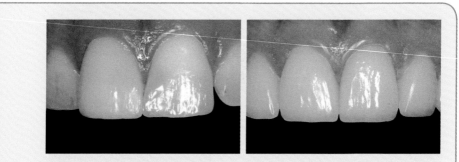

This dentist wanted a more uniform, symmetrical look. Notice how natural his one crown and veneers look. Your teeth should look as though they're growing out of the gums.

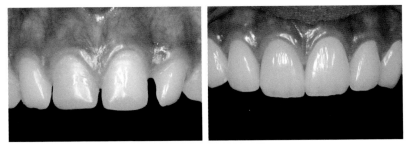

BEFORE   AFTER

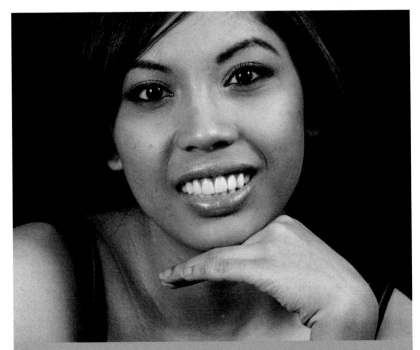

Rizza wanted to close her spaces and whiten her teeth. Notice the surface texture and ridging that mimick natural teeth.

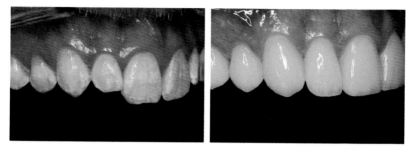

BEFORE   AFTER

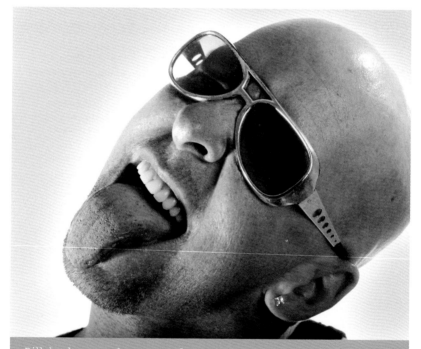

Bill had wanted veneers for 20 years to cover his discolored teeth. Here he is rocking out his new smile. Again, notice how natural the veneers look.

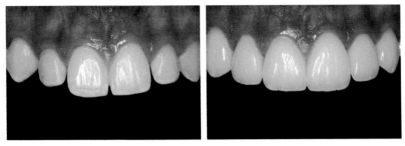

BEFORE   AFTER

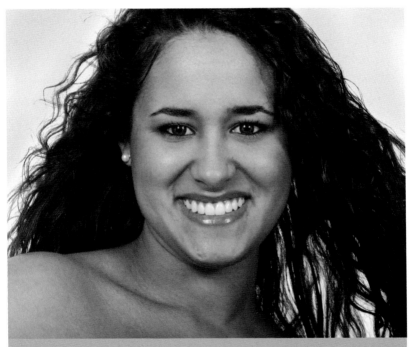

Notice the translucency and texture of these veneers. You can't detect where the veneer begins or ends because each is shaped the way teeth naturally look. The veneers are not bright white, opaque blocks of porcelain that don't even resemble teeth.

Concern or Myth #3: "My dentist told me veneers don't work."

Now, why would dentists say veneers don't work? Perhaps because they are uncomfortable doing them. Perhaps they tried a couple of times and had bad results or couldn't please their patients. Rather than admitting their failure and spending time and money learning how to do it correctly, they just copped out and declared that veneers don't work. I say, get another opinion—fast! We hear it so many times: A patient needed to have a veneer replaced or wanted to have a veneer placed, and the dentist claims veneers won't work in this situation and decides to aggressively prepare the tooth for a crown instead. Then the weakened tooth breaks, needs to be removed, and must be replaced with an implant. All because that dentist didn't care to keep current with today's advancements in conservative dentistry.

How Many Veneers Do I Need?

This number depends on both your goals and your budget. For a person wanting a "smile makeover," we recommend eight to 14 veneers depending on how many teeth show in your smile. Six is a very common number of veeners done by untrained dentists. But six veneers should not be done very often, unless the patient is not wanting to go much whiter and the next four teeth in the smile are very prominent, so the six veneers will just blend right in. We often see patients come in unhappy with six veneers, and it's extremely obvious why. The front six are bright white and stick out further. They simply don't go with the rest of the person's smile, so it just looks "off" or fake. Doing at least

eight or as many as 14 lets the patient make the changes he or
she wants (perhaps whiter, longer, sexier, or whatever) without
looking like it doesn't fit. Budget usually determines how many
we do. Some people may want 10 or 12 because that's what
really shows in a big smile; however, their budget only allows
for eight. Most patients can get away with eight and they can
always come back and do a few more when their budget allows;
matching back teeth is usually pretty easy to do.

Whether a person does just top teeth or both top and bottom also depends, again on goals and budget. If budget is not
an issue and a person is unhappy with his or her bottom teeth,
then veneer the lower teeth, usually eight to 10 veneers. If a
person's bottom teeth are fairly straight and white and he or
she is happy with them, then just do the top teeth—as long as
the person's bite, or the way the teeth come together, allows it.
(See the later section on full mouth rehabilitation to read more
about why some people need to do both top and bottom teeth.)

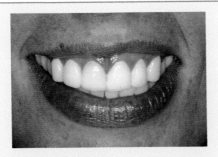

Christine came to see us, unhappy with the way her smile looked
after having her general, "cosmetic" dentist place six veneers. Her
complaint was that they appeared fake, bulky, and opaque. We
agree. These do not even resemble what teeth look like naturally.
And doing just six makes them jump out even more.

Again, some patients will do their tops first, then do the lowers when their budget allows.

Finally, some people have great smiles except for maybe one or two or even four teeth. It is possible to veneer just that one or those few teeth to match and blend right in with the other teeth. We typically recommend that the patient whiten his or her teeth first, so we can match the new whiter smile. This is probably one of the hardest treatments we perform today, matching one veneer to the rest of the teeth. Our goal is to mimic nature. We explain to our patients that it may take a few visits to get it just

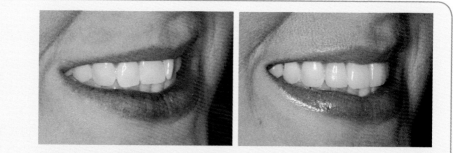

BEFORE   AFTER

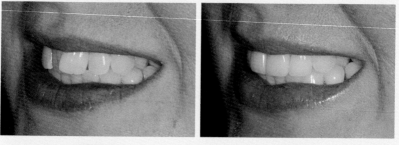

BEFORE   AFTER

Christina couldn't afford eight veneers for a full smile makeover, so we just did four veneers to correct the crowding and made the veneers blend in with her other teeth.

right. When we try in veneers, whether it's one or 20, we always allow the patient to stand up and view them in four or five different mirrors and lighting arrangements to make sure everything looks great. "I don't like the way they look" is a common thing we hear when we see an unhappy cosmetic patient, and we ask, why did you let the dentist cement them in if you didn't like it? And patients often reply that either they didn't get a chance to see before the veneers were cemented in or they had to look while lying back in the chair and couldn't really tell. So always make sure you look at the veneers first, before they are bonded into

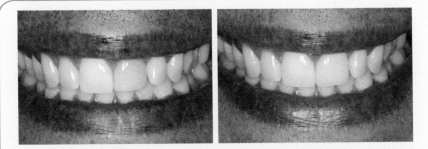

BEFORE   AFTER

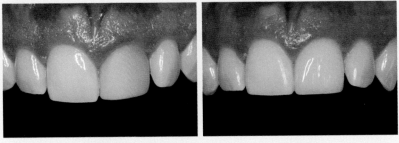

BEFORE   AFTER

Michael wanted only one veneer to replace bonding that another dentist had done for him. He wanted it to look natural and blend in with his other teeth.

place, to make sure you love them, because once you get home, it's too late. To cut them off and redo them is like starting over.

What to Know about Color

The final color of a veneer is composed of four different things:

- the tooth itself, which is the canvas;
- the cement that bonds the porcelain to the tooth;
- the ingot composed of the pressed porcelain; and
- the layering porcelain that's laid on top of the ingot for natural results.

The color of the veneer will be graduated from the biting edge to the gum line, like natural teeth. In natural teeth, the most saturation of color is at the gum line. This is because the dentin from the tooth shows through to the surface enamel. Often with crowns and veneers, the final result is too mono-chromatic (one color). This fake look becomes a tip-off that the tooth is artificial. Another clue: The extra thickness at the gum line doesn't allow for the ingot to press thin and become more translucent, thus allowing more underlying tooth color to come through.

You should have a chance to test-drive your smile while wearing temporaries so you can decide what looks best on your face. Of course, ask for feedback from your family and friends. It's funny, but most often when our clients look at their new smiles for the first time, they're shocked and want the final veneers to be toned down a bit in color. But then we receive a phone call from them a few days later, and they're exclaiming they love the color. It can take several days to get used to your new look.

Have you noticed that society continually pushes the white smile limits? That is, what society deems to be natural-looking white teeth today is 10 shades whiter than it was a decade ago. Yes, it's possible to get a natural look that's white, even by today's standards, but it creates a unique challenge because it's not acceptable to have a fake-looking smile. Veneers have gotten a bad rap because the teeth often look too big for the face or too white or just plain wrong. The color must match the person's complexion; the shapes must go with the person's overall image and complement the color; the smile has to match the person's personality. It takes the eye of a stylist to understand the intimate relationship among beauty, fashion, and smiles.

What to Know about Fashion

It seems a bit silly to say this, but a dentist working on smiles needs to inherently understand what looks good. After all, the dentist's taste is a big part of designing your veneers.

When you go to interview a dentist, can you get a feel for whether he or she has good fashion sense? The dentist may not have the same idea as you do of what looks good. Therefore, if you don't think you're on the same fashion wavelength, it's going to be difficult to get what you want for your teeth.

For example, would you get fashion advice from a stylist who wears inappropriate clothing? Would you get your hair cut by a stylist whose hairdo is 20 years out of style? Would you get your teeth done by a dentist whose teeth are ugly? Of course not! Just because we're health care practitioners doesn't mean we're exempt from having good taste. Again, we hear it often: A patient comes to us in the middle of their cosmetic treatment, wanting a second opinion. The patient has been in temporaries for months and claims the dentist has tried in a number of restorations and none look good, even though the dentist says it looks great. The patient shouldn't have to tell the dentist when something doesn't look right.

So take it all in, from the moment you walk through the door to the moment you leave, and evaluate whether this dentist can be trusted with what will look good on your face.

What to Know about the Four-Visit Process

The smile makeover procedure, from start to finish, takes four visits over six to eight weeks.

First Visit: The fast and easy one. The dentist will ready your pre-op records, including x-rays, photos, and impressions, and give you a full exam. You can also further discuss your goals and concerns. If a dentist doesn't take these important steps, he or she is not serious about designing your smile correctly. Why? Because the lab needs this information to design your smile in wax and make templates that will be used in the second visit. *Note:* In some cases a wax-up is not needed and the dentist may do a mock-up which means he designs your smile first in the office and uses that new design for the template for your temps.)

Time of visit: one to one and a half hours.

Second Visit: Longer and more difficult because it involves numbing and drilling. But it's also exciting because you get your temporaries at the end, and they look awesome! Some clients even take a sedative to help them relax through this visit, and this seems to make time fly.

You'd typically wear your temporaries for about three weeks to test-drive them. Do you love both the color and the shapes? Remember, you can make changes that differ from your temporaries. That way, your dentist and lab can communicate your wants and predictably create your veneers after this template. (See boxed *Post-Op Instructions after the Second Visit* on pages 42–43.)

Time of visit: two to five hours, depending on number of teeth being addressed.

Third Visit: Try on and cement your new veneers. Take this opportunity to get a good look at your new smile before it's permanently cemented in. *This is super important.* When new patients come in unhappy with their veneers, I ask if they told their dentist before the veneers were bonded in. Far too often, they reply that the dentist just bonded them in without giving them the opportunity to check out the new veneers. That's crazy! Make sure you get a good look *first,* because once they're in, they're in.

Time of visit: two to four hours, depending on how many teeth and the complexity of the job.

Fourth Visit: Post-op visit to double check everything, such as making sure your bite is correct, and address any concerns. We also have a big photo shoot to really let you show off your new smile!

Time of visit: 30 to 60 minutes.

Treating TMD

Sometimes people experience a more serious type of misalignment involving the jaw. The temporomandibular joint (TMJ) is

Post-Op Instructions after the Second Visit

People often have questions about how to take care of their temporaries, so here are a few things we tell our clients. (Your dentist may have different instructions depending on your procedure and an individual approach.)

- Avoid eating hard foods or anything chewy.
- Although your temporaries are designed to be a model for your definitive restorations, they will not feel like your final restorations, which will be smoother and more life-like in appearance.
- Your teeth may be sensitive to temperature and chewing with your temporaries, but this will subside after your final restorations are placed.
- Some patients experience a sensation of contraction and tightness with cold or hot food or beverages.
- You will have some discomfort after your preparation appointment. The sensitivity that patients experience varies. This initial discomfort is relieved in most cases by taking 600 mg of Ibuprofen every six hours as needed, not to exceed 3,200 mg in a 24-hour period. If your sensitivity can't be managed with Ibuprofen, please call your dentist and/or follow your dentist's instructions.

the joint that connects the lower jaw to the skull and allows the jaw to open and close. Any problem with the joint is referred to as TMD, or temporomandibular disorder. Many people have been told they clench and/or grind their teeth at night. Tooth grinding is also called "bruxism," which can become a subconscious habit during sleep. However, it can occur during the day as well as at nighttime. People may notice it at certain times of the day, their spouse may tell them they can hear them grind at night, or a dentist may be the first one to tell them. A variety of reasons cause people to grind, including an abnormal bite,

- It's extremely important to keep your gums as healthy as possible between your preparation and cementation appointments. The following regimen is essential:
  - You'll be given hydrogen peroxide syringes (which are refillable) that should be used at the gum line of your temporaries three to four times daily until your next appointment. Switch to the light green solution (Chlorhexidine) about one week before your next appointment to bond in your new veneers.
  - If you had laser gum therapy performed, use the rubber tip stimulator very gently under the gums two to three times a day for the first week.
  - Bridge threaders are provided to use between your temporaries. These are pieces of floss that have a stiff end to help thread through the temporaries and are connected for strength. The temporary veneers can't be flossed in the usual way for these few weeks.
- If your bite feels "high" after the anesthetic wears off, please call for an adjustment. Over time, a high temporary will bruise the ligament around the tooth and may cause it to become sensitive.

stress, or even genetics. Stress can make the jaw clench and grind, causing TMD and myofacial pain.

Facial muscles, jaw joints, upper and lower jaws, and teeth must fit together and function in balance for proper chewing to occur. A bite that's misaligned causes damage to the joints, muscles, and teeth. If the bite is not addressed, people risk breaking and wearing down their natural teeth as well as their existing dental work. This wear can occur in many different patterns and may involve only the back teeth, only the front teeth, or in some cases, all the teeth. Then facial muscles can become strained and overworked, causing extreme pain in a person's head and neck areas. People who have migraines and headaches often seek out their physician for a solution, but they'd be well advised to also check with their dentist.

Misalignment can show up in several ways, including injury to the jaw, arthritis in the jaw joint, missing teeth, teeth that have shifted, crooked teeth that are misaligned, or ill-fitting dental work. Many variables and factors go into diagnosing and treating TMJ issues, with no black-and-white answer easily found. Some people have a bite that's "off" or wrong, yet they never show any signs of joint issues or tooth wear; others can't tolerate any discrepancy.

Signs and symptoms include sensitive, broken, worn-down, or loose teeth; difficulty chewing or opening your mouth when eating and yawning; clicking and popping of your jaw joint; sore, stiff muscles when you wake up in the mornings; and frequent headaches.

Sometimes, in severe cases, surgery of the joint is needed—typically a last resort when none of the other treatments have helped. Ways to treat TMJ issues range widely, depending on the people involved as well as their goals for their teeth and smile. Their bite can be improved by reshaping or equilibrating their teeth, or by having their teeth repositioned through either orthodontics or a full mouth rehab using veneers and crowns.

A night guard or appliance may be used by itself or in combination with other treatments. Guards can typically decrease the problem by helping to protect the teeth from grinding and reducing the damage, but they rarely cure the issue. Over-the-counter night guards won't do the job, because the guard needs to be fitted properly and equilibrated to work well. If you need a guard, talk with your dentist to obtain one and have it fitted.

Another adjunct used to help with TMJ problems is Botox,

which is used to decrease the force of certain muscles. Botox can help with headaches, decrease biting force, and slim down square, large jaw lines.

What your dentist recommends depends on training and experience in treating TMJ problems.

Not every dentist knows how to diagnose and treat complex cases of TMD—and maybe not even the simple cases. That's why it's important to research the right dentist for you.

Beware: This can be confusing. A client came to us after having a full mouth rehab with someone else just the week before. She was unhappy with the way it turned out and needed to find someone to *redo* part of it. She had asked dentist friends for advice and researched online. She got quite confused. Some sources said see a "Pankey" dentist, or a dentist trained by Dawson; others said see an "LVI doc" or a "PAC-live grad"; and the list went on and on.

Several schools of thought exist on this topic in the dental field. Although for a while tension reigned among proponents of the different philosophies, I feel everyone began to realize that the different methods can all work fine in certain situations and perhaps we can learn from one another. It's not necessarily where the dentist trained (the teaching institution) or the philosophy that's important, but the skill, talent, intuition, and range of knowledge of a particular dentist.

So what's the answer? Dentists have several ways to diagnose and treat these problems, and I can't say which way is best for you. I *will* tell you to have a conversation with all dentists you're interviewing and ask about their education, experience, and technologies.

Great technology is now available to help these cases go smoothly and last a long time, but equipment for this can be expensive, so not every dentist has it. Make sure your dentist has special instruments to measure your joint before and after treatment (such as a JVA or Doppler), as well as a computer sensor such as a T-scan to measure your bite. I suggest you see several dentists and find out whom you connect with best. Make sure you evaluate the work each dentist does and examine the results he or she has had.

Full Mouth Rehab

Some people may wish to enhance only the teeth that show in their smile, but may have occlusion or bite issues that prevent them from doing just that.

These cases require a full mouth rehabilitation, in which the entire mouth is redone to create optimal positions for the teeth and the way they bite or come together. This overhaul—sometimes called a "dental facelift"—can correct years of wear and tear on the teeth and take years off their appearance.

A full mouth rehab typically involves all the teeth and is accomplished with veneers and crowns. (We don't get too caught up in distinguishing between the two; we use whichever will be best cosmetically, as well as functionally.) Typically this is done in two phases; the first phase takes place in five visits (about eight weeks), and the second phase in two visits (about four weeks). Total time is about three months from start to finish. Here's how the procedure flows.

First Visit: The dentist takes x-rays, pictures, and impressions to be sent to the lab for the ceramist to create the ideal smile and bite out of wax. We will also make a custom guard to wear at night so we can record the bite (how teeth come together) on the next visit.

Time of visit: one and a half hours.

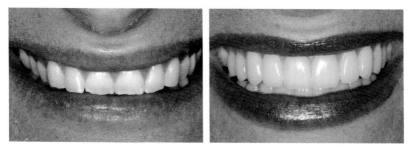

BEFORE AFTER

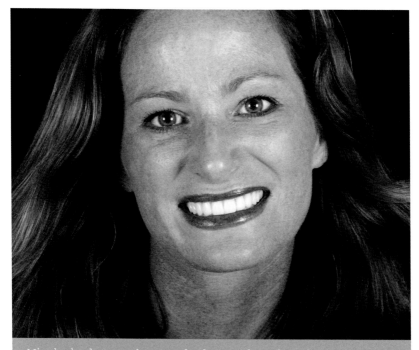

Nicole had worn her teeth down, changing the appearance of not only her teeth but her entire face. We gave her twenty veneers and restored her smile, her facial appearance, and her confidence.

Porcelain Veneers — Frequently Asked Questions

How long will my veneers last?
Veneers can last anywhere from 10 to 20 years or more, depending on each person. Your bite has a lot to do with how long they will last. Your dentist should let you know during your exam. What options you have will help extend the life of your veneers. They include wearing a bite guard while you sleep or veneering more teeth to control the bite. Also, your hygiene, home care, and medical conditions will affect the lifespan of your dental work.

Can I still get cavities?
Areas covered by the porcelain cannot get cavities, but you can still get cavities on other parts of your teeth. We recommend cleanings every six months or more frequently so that cavities are caught when they are small and can be filled without needing to replace a veneer.

Will my veneers stain?
Your veneers will not stain like natural teeth.

How many appointments will it take to get my veneers?
A typical schedule for getting veneers consists of three to eight appointments spread out over six to 12 weeks, depending on the extent of the work needed.

How much will my veneers cost?
The cost of veneers depends on the number of teeth that need to be included to improve your smile. We typically charge fees based on the case as a whole and take into account all the treatments required to get the best final results. A good ball-park figure is $1,200 to $2,500 per tooth, depending on the city and the dentist.

Will I have to be careful what I eat?
You can eat anything you would normally eat with your regular teeth, including apples. Remember, veneers are not

super-strong teeth or stronger than natural teeth, so we rec-ommend that if you normally eat ice or jaw breakers—or open beer bottles with your teeth— then *change your habits for good*. Habits that can damage your natural teeth can certainly damage your new veneers.

Does getting veneers hurt my teeth?

Find a dentist who practices conservative techniques for por-celain veneers. Most of the time, the veneers are entirely in the outer enamel of your teeth. The veneers provided should not weaken your teeth or make them more prone to fracture. Patients rarely need anything other than a mild painkiller for dis-comfort. It's also unlikely to require a root canal from a veneer. That said, if you are having old silver fillings replaced at the same time or have large cavities being fixed with the veneers, then the chance of post-operative pain or the need for a root canal does increase.

Will my veneers ever pop off?

A properly bonded veneer will not pop off your teeth. A veneer can fracture from too much stress, but a whole veneer should not just come off.

Will my veneer ever break?

Veneers can chip or break like natural teeth when subjected to eating stress. Most of the time, stress situations are caught before a problem emerges, by using computerized bite-taking technology. Veneers can also get craze lines, much like natural teeth when subjected to biting forces. Properly bonded veneers will not pop off the tooth, even when they are fractured in half.

What are the most frequent complications with getting veneers?

Complications with veneers most often occur while the patient is wearing temporaries. The back teeth are usually prepared the most conservatively, and the temporary veneer can pop off dur-ing eating. This does not happen with the permanent veneers. Remember, temporaries provide a chance to try out the look and bite of your new smile, because they closely resemble your

continued on next page

continued from previous page

porcelain veneers. From time to time, a temporary veneer does break or come off. We have developed a system for you to fix the emergency at home so that you never go around looking bad. Discuss this with your dentists so you know you'll be taken care of in the event of an emergency.

Porcelain veneers stand out as one of the greatest advancements of dentistry because they make it possible to transform the worst of smiles into gorgeous ones. It's one way to truly achieve a "wow" smile if you were not born with one. But this extremely technique-sensitive procedure requires a talented, well-trained dentist, so again, do your research before investing several thousands of dollars in a new smile.

Second Visit: Takes place one to two weeks after the first visit to record the bite. You will need to wear your custom guard all night and morning until you see us. We'll be the first ones to take it out, because we don't want your teeth to touch. You'll come back about three weeks later.

Time of visit: 30 minutes.

Third Visit: You are numbed and your teeth are conservatively reshaped; an impression of them is taken for the lab. (Some patients take a sedative to help them relax and pass the time. We also have movies and music to entertain you during the procedure.) You will leave that day with your new (temporary) smile. You get to test-drive your new smile in temporaries to make sure you love the color and shapes! The porcelain veneers take approximately three weeks to create in the lab.

Time of visit: three to six hours.

Fourth Visit: To cement in your new veneers, we numb the area while we take off your temporaries and try on your veneers with different-colored cements. They must meet your approval before we permanently cement them to your teeth. (You may want to take a sedative for this visit, too.)

Time of visit: two to five hours.

Fifth Visit: For a final cleanup and check-in to see if there is anything sharp or areas you have trouble flossing. We check your bite and take some post-op photos. We will also take impressions of your back teeth for the next visit.

Time of visit: one hour.

Sixth Visit: About three weeks later, you are numbed again and we prepare your back teeth. You'll leave with temporaries on your back teeth.

Time of visit: three hours.

Seventh Visit: The dentist removes your temps and puts in your new back crowns. You will be numb for this visit, too.

Time of visit: two hours.

Final Visit and Photo Shoot: Time to show off your new smile!

Time of visit: one hour.

Patient Expectations

One of the hardest jobs we have is managing our patients' expectations. Every case is different, as is every outcome. We try to be very realistic about what we are going to accomplish and what, if any, compromises might be necessary. This helps us minimize disappointment and often helps us exceed patient expectations.

Meeting expectations often hinges on the communication between the dentist and the patient. Chapter 8 discusses in detail how to research your smile makeover dentist, but I thought it was appropriate to touch on it here since porcelain veneers are both the most dramatic of treatments, as well as the treatment that varies the most between dentists. I am familiar with doing consultations with frustrated patients who feel like their dentists have given up too easily on making them happy with their new smiles. It is common to get frustrated when you are unable to get your desired smile from a dentist who does not typically provide excellent cosmetics. This also causes the dentists frustration, because they feel like they are providing their best treatment, but it is still not the smile you had in mind. You want to choose a dentist who is confident, yet realistic when discussing your smile and your goals. You want a dentist who listens to your concerns, who will take the time to explain potential compromises, and who will try everything he or she can to make you happy.

Chapter 3
Treatments and Myths of Teeth Whitening

Teeth whitening is the most requested cosmetic dental procedure in the world. People want teeth as white as possible without looking fake. However, they now consider a "natural" white to be many shades lighter than what people considered to be natural 10 years ago. Patients' demands are pushing the limits of what society will tolerate.

Whitening is easy, conservative, and inexpensive—if done with integrity. If you love everything but the color of your teeth, whitening may be just the right procedure for you to greatly enhance your smile. The right dentist will help you determine whether you're a good candidate for teeth whitening.

Depending on your budget and lifestyle, you have several options. You can have your teeth whitened approximately eight shades in about an hour with an in-office whitening treatment. Or you can wear professional, take-home teeth-whitening trays, provided by your dentist, during the day or overnight. You can also buy whitening products at the drug-store, but these aren't as effective, and they involve risks addressed later in this chapter.

Are you a good candidate for teeth whitening? The answer depends on the dental work you've already had and the kind of teeth you have. Teeth discolored from tetracycline or too much fluoride may bleach unevenly; healthy yellow teeth respond best to tooth-whitening products; dark gray, brown, and black hues are more difficult to whiten. If your teeth are any of these darker colors, you must be persistent and consistently use take-home trays for several months to achieve decent results.

Keep in mind that only natural tooth structure will whiten, while veneers, crowns, and bonding remain their original color.

Why Do Teeth Discolor?

Genetics may be the cause of tooth discoloration. Some people naturally have white teeth, while others have dark-colored teeth that don't bleach well. Generally, teeth look darker with age as the dentin layer becomes thicker. Trauma may also cause a tooth or teeth to darken over time.

Discoloration can be caused by smoking as well as by drinking and eating stain-causing beverages and foods such as coffee, tea, red wine, tomato sauce, and soy sauce. Your dentist may initially be able to polish away these superficial stains, but after a while, they may penetrate and stain the actual tooth structure. Some medications, such as tetracycline, can discolor teeth. Silver fillings may make a tooth appear gray. Fluoride can cause various effects, such as internal gray, brown, or black staining or banding on the teeth. Be aware of all these possibilities.

So if you have a mixture of natural and restored teeth, after you whiten, you may need to have the synthetic parts replaced to match your new, lighter color. Consult with your dentist, who can assist you with what will work best for your smile.

Whitening Methods Explained

Several whitening methods are available. Let's look at the advantages and disadvantages of each of the following and how they work.

- Take-home trays
- In-office whitening
- Over-the-counter treatments

Take-Home Trays: We love take-home trays. Our experience has proven they give the best results, and the process is easy. First, your dentist will take impressions of your top and bottom teeth to make clear, custom whitening trays that fit comfortably over each arch. Your dentist or dental team member will have you insert the trays before you leave to ensure they fit well. The tray should fit intimately with the teeth, without any gaping or rocking.

If you have older trays at home and plan to buy new bleach, ask your dentist to check the fit before you begin whitening. You want to make sure that your trays haven't distorted or that your teeth haven't shifted so the trays no longer fit well.

Your dentist or dental team member will show you how to insert whitening gel in the tray for each tooth being whitened. Remember, less is more. You don't need to pour in a lot of bleach; a tiny amount does the trick. You'll find directions included with the bleach, showing the exact amount.

Remember in science class when a drop of water was placed between two slides, and it spread to cover a much larger surface? Same thing happens here. As the peroxide breaks down, oxygen enters the enamel and dentin to lighten discolorations. The structure of the tooth isn't changed—only the color, which becomes lighter. People usually notice results after the first or second application, with maximum results generally occurring after five to 14 days of treatment.

Different types of bleaching gel are available to dentists for their patients to use. Some are worn overnight while others "do the trick" in 30 minutes. We find our clients prefer the shorter-acting gels because of their convenience.

You have to be both consistent and persistent when you commit to the whitening treatment, doing it for the recommended number of days to achieve satisfactory results. Since it typically takes 10 to 14 days for optimal results, plan ahead if you're whitening your teeth to be ready for an upcoming event.

Also know that everyone experiences a different degree of sensitivity with this process; some people can whiten with no problem, while others experience some pain. If you're ultra-sensitive, you may find it difficult to continue to whiten for up to two weeks. Possible options are to skip days, whiten for shorter time intervals, or request fluoride to supplement—or use the in-office method described next. For reasons of compliance and sensitivity, it's important to discuss whitening with your dentist and determine which method will work best for you.

In-office Whitening or Power Bleaching: The most intense, fastest way to whiten teeth is by power bleaching in the dentist's office. You can likely choose from a number of in-office systems that are similar to one another. The one your dentist uses depends on his or her education and experience.

Expect the procedure to take about an hour. We suggest you bring an iPod or ask your dentist if you can watch TV to help pass the time.

Before undergoing the procedure, be sure to have your teeth evaluated by the dentist for whitening effectiveness. Most often, we recommend take-home trays as an adjunct to in-office whitening for optimal results. Although in-office whitening is effective and fast, it rarely gets a person's teeth as white as bleaching with take-home trays.

During this process, retractors are placed in your mouth to keep your lips away from the bleach and the light that's used for the whitening. Your gums are isolated from your teeth using a special material that blocks out tissue that may be harmed by the concentrated bleach. If a light is used with the whitening system, you have to wear special glasses that filter out the UV light from the lamp.

Once the isolating process is completed, the bleach is placed on the top and bottom teeth. Systems may vary a little, but usually you receive three 15-minute applications of bleach. At the end of the three application sessions, a liquid fluoride is placed on the teeth to decrease the amount of postoperative sensitivity. Some patients experience sensitivity with this procedure, but it lasts less than 24 hours. Others experience no sensitivity.

A UV lamp is an important part of the Zoom! whitening experience, but several in-office treatments are available that whiten without a light. Results of studies on the efficacy of using a UV lamp range from negligible improvements to slight improvements when light assists the whitening process. How do you decide? Consider the dentist's experience and results, whether or not a lamp is used. Rest assured, the UV light won't hurt your teeth, and it just may improve results.

Experience has shown that dehydration of the teeth immediately after whitening interferes with an accurate assessment of the post-whitening shade. For this reason, it's best for dentists to evaluate the shade change a couple of days after the treatment.

The negatives associated with in-office whitening are cost (it is more expensive than the take-home trays) and fairly short-term results. The procedure creates a whitening result that lasts anywhere from three months to two years, depending on the patient's home care and lifestyle. We recommend getting take-home trays to maintain your new shade simply by whitening once a month for 15 to 30 minutes.

Summary of In-office vs. Take-home Procedures

- The in-office procedure takes about one hour, while the tray system takes 10 to14 days to reach optimal results.
- You may experience less sensitivity with in-office whitening, because you have only 24 hours of sensitivity (if you have any) versus a possible two weeks of sensitivity with the trays.
- One hour of in-office whitening may provide only a boost toward your new, whiter smile. Whitening with take-home trays allows for greater flexibility in achieving your whitening goals.
- The in-office procedure costs more than the take-home trays. Prices vary across the country, but the price range of trays is $100–$400 and the price range of in-office whitening is $500–$1,200. Again, do your research. Don't automatically use the lowest-priced dentist, or you may be unhappy with the results.
- Discuss your options with a well-informed dentist to see which would be ideal for you.

Professional vs. Over-the-Counter (OTC) Treatments

Whitening toothpastes and over-the-counter whiteners are effective for some people. These products are weaker and less expensive than those used by dentists and can be used without the supervision of the dental team. However, the results are less dramatic and often don't last as long.

Over-the-counter products come in various concentrations and delivery modalities. They usually contain a low concentration of hydrogen peroxide, and their advertising claims may not be proven by research. However, the Crest Whitestrips system by Procter & Gamble is backed by a number of clinical studies that prove it whitens teeth in some situations. We tell clients that **whitening strips** are worth a try, plus we can help them achieve more substantial results if they're dissatisfied with using the strips.

Consumer Reports alerts consumers to the fact that **whitening toothpastes** do not change the color of teeth. It also notes that many advertise effectiveness without data to substantiate their claims. Whitening toothpastes only scrub away surface stains with abrasives in the paste. Although a few toothpastes on the market include forms of hydrogen peroxide, it's not concentrated enough, and contact time with the teeth isn't long enough, to produce measurable results. We encourage you not

Follow Instructions!

In our experience, following instructions is always the biggest issue when whitening teeth. Even if a system has been proven effective, it won't work well—or work at all—if a person doesn't use it as instructed.

to select your toothpaste brand based on potential whitening results, but to look for ingredients that help keep your mouth, teeth, and dental work healthy.

Other over-the-counter whiteners use one-size-fits-all **whitening trays** that don't, in fact, fit *anybody* well. These trays result in the whitening gel being diluted and washed away by saliva, and the peroxide in the gel is more likely to irritate and burn the gums.

Beware of over-the-counter gimmicks that promise fast whitening times (and compare them to professional whiteners) as well as those that come with their own versions of **whitening lights**. Save these types of lights for use in the kitchen when the power goes out!

The Bleaching Process

Bleaching When You Have Sensitive Teeth

Getting an in-office whitening treatment is the best choice for highly sensitive teeth. If you have areas of your teeth that are more sensitive than others, such as pockets of gum recession, we can block them out with our liquid dam material to protect them. Then the sensitivity usually lasts up to 24 hours, and you can take over-the-counter pain relievers during that time. If you become sensitive during the procedure, we might use local anesthetic to numb the teeth during whitening, just as you'd have any other body part anesthetized before having a cosmetic procedure.

Before coming in for your whitening, switch to sensitivity-protection toothpaste for two or three weeks. Or, if necessary, we can prescribe a stronger toothpaste that seals the dental tubules and makes the teeth less susceptible to sensitivity.

Questions that Address Myths and Concerns about Whitening

Does the light used in in-office treatments really do anything?

Manufacturers claim that application of laser UV or halogen activates the bleaching material through photoinitiators in the whitening gel to enhance its effectiveness and accelerate the bleaching process. The effectiveness of light is controversial. A few studies support the use of light, but other studies find little value while noting increased sensitivity. We use the Zoom! system in our office because clients most commonly request this system. We've also used a non-light system called Opalescence, which produced results that were nearly the same. Variations were due to the clients' teeth, not the system. Some people's teeth are resistant to whitening regardless of the system or the length of time the teeth are processed. If a client's teeth don't whiten well, we suggest using trays to continue the whitening at home.

Does whitening hurt the integrity of your teeth?

No. Whitening works because peroxide chemically changes the structure of staining molecules in the enamel and dentin. The inorganic and organic makeup of the tooth remains unchanged. The pH of most professional bleaches used is neutral in order to control sensitivity and will not erode teeth.

Can you bleach your teeth if they are sensitive?

Yes. However, teeth whitening is a cosmetic procedure to improve your looks; most cosmetic procedures include some discomfort, and whitening is not necessarily an exception to that rule. Expect some sensitivity as a possible side effect to achieving final whitening results.

Does the whitening gel hurt your gums?

The gel used is meant for teeth, not gums, and the bleach in the gel can burn your gums if it comes in contact with them for long enough. It may turn your gums white, but this is not permanent and typically goes away in 15–30 minutes. Your dentist can prevent this during in-office treatment. If you're using in-home trays, be careful to use the specified amount of gel.

If you're highly sensitive, we can make your whitening trays ahead of time. You'd use them to apply fluoride gels at home for 30 minutes a day for a week before your whitening appointment. *Note:* Dental fluorosis, a condition that discolors the teeth, is caused by using too much fluoride in early childhood when teeth are forming. However, fluorosis is not a problem with mature teeth.

How Bleaching Works

The basic bleaching process works by oxidizing the organic colored material within the tooth, reducing its color intensity. The process doesn't weaken the structure of teeth, but it can cause some sensitivity.

The most commonly used agents in the bleaching process are hydrogen peroxide and carbamide peroxide. Carbamide peroxide breaks down to hydrogen peroxide and urea, and the hydrogen peroxide further breaks down to water and oxygen. The peroxide diffuses through the enamel into the dentin, where it has the greatest effect on the color change of the tooth. A higher concentration of peroxide achieves faster results. You can expect similar final results from products with less concentration if you increase the frequency of application or contact time.

Maintain the White

How long your whitening results last depends on your genetics and lifestyle. During the whitening process at home, avoid eating discoloring foods and drinking beverages that might stain your teeth. Also avoid acidic foods and beverages to manage sensitivity. Remember to always brush gently and use a soft toothbrush. Establish a regular cleaning schedule with your dentist or hygienist to remove surface stains.

Most of our clients ask for the in-office Zoom! procedure and get the trays made at the same appointment. The in-office procedure whitens by eight to 10 shades, while using the tray at home continues the whitening process for three to 10 days. The trays can then be used monthly to maintain the whitening effect you want.

Results to Expect from Whitening

Our goals for whitening are to whiten your teeth as much as possible and maintain that whiteness. We've found that most people want really white teeth, but we don't want to go over-board or they won't look natural. A small percentage of people naturally have bright white teeth, and this is what most people want to achieve. Our recommendations are based on that goal.

In most cases, teeth will whiten only so much. When we create veneers, we stress a natural look, making the veneers mimic real teeth. *They can still look natural if done well.* When whitening natural teeth, we try to get them as white as the patient wants, which is usually as white as they can get. Even if they're a bright white, they rarely look fake because they *are* real teeth.

You can whiten your teeth with trays alone, but that takes longer and teeth become more sensitive, so application compliance goes down. Result? Your whitest smile may never be achieved. Some people don't want to be bothered with trays at all, so they have the in-office procedure every six months when they have their teeth cleaned.

In-office or dentist-supplied take-home whiteners aim to get your teeth eight to 10 shades whiter. To some people, this appears to be a dramatic change, yet others may find this degree of change disappointing. For example, if your teeth start at the bottom of the shade guide and they're whitened eight shades, they'll only reach the middle of the guide. It's an improvement, but your teeth will still be far from white. On the other hand, if you start with fairly light teeth and bleach them eight shades, they'll appear bright white. Have the dentist help you manage this process. Be sure to convey your expectations so you won't be disappointed in the result.

For people who want dramatic results, it's often necessary to get porcelain veneers, which can be made just about any shade of whiteness you desire.

We've seen many clients who've spent hundreds, even thousands of dollars trying to whiten their teeth, but their teeth just didn't bleach well. They come to us to see if there's *anything* else we can do. At this point, we discuss using veneers to achieve the level of white they want.

The Effects of Stains and Discoloration

The white you can achieve may be limited by genetic and lifestyle factors, which play a major role in the color of your teeth. Stains that discolor your teeth can be caused by any of the following:

- Foods and beverages—Berries, soy sauce, coffee, tea, cola, red wine, etc.
- Fluoride—White spots known as "calcifications."
- Smoking—Yellow or brown stains from nicotine.
- Heredity—Naturally brighter enamel and dentin respond well to whitening.
- Antibiotics—Tetracycline taken during childhood turns teeth blue, brown, or gray and typically makes them unresponsive to whitening.
- Trauma—Resulting in a lone dark tooth, which can be bleached from the inside or covered with a veneer.

Post-Whitening Procedure Instructions

After the in-office procedure, we recommended you avoid smoking and taking in dark-staining foods and drinks—such as coffee, tea, red wine, mustard, ketchup, soy sauce, red sauce, and berry sauce—for 48 hours. Also avoid drinking sodas and citrus-containing beverages such as orange juice for a couple of days to prevent greater sensitivity. Be sure to brush and floss consistently.

Teeth can appear to have white spots after bleaching, which is normal, and they typically go away after several days. Some people's teeth have white spots *before* they bleach. These spots tend to worsen (that is, they get even whiter) after bleaching, but the contrast subsides after a few days.

Bleach is meant for teeth only, not gums. Burning the gums from the bleach is a common complaint and can occur with any whitening treatment, but it's certainly avoidable. If you're bleaching at home, make sure you don't put too much bleach in your tray, because the excess can ooze out and burn your gums.

Realize that over-the-counter treatments are not custom-fit to your mouth, so the tray or strip may extend onto your gums, causing them to burn. By contrast, during an in-office treatment, your teeth are isolated and your gums are completely covered to avoid this. But don't worry if you experience a bit of burning; it doesn't cause irreversible damage. The gums may burn or ache for a few hours and may even turn white, but these effects go away fairly quickly.

Now that you have the information you need to help you make an informed decision about whitening your teeth, discuss your situation with your dentist.

Ready to discuss procedures for straightening your teeth? Let's move on to the next chapter.

✳

Chapter 4

Invisalign and Other Ways to Straighten Teeth

Good news: Braces aren't just for kids anymore!

Having straight teeth is important for both cosmetic and health advantages. The most common reasons for needing braces are to correct a "bad bite," straighten crooked or crowded teeth, and close spaces or gaps. Having crooked teeth or a bad bite can affect your ability to keep your teeth clean because it's more difficult to floss. Crooked teeth can even cause headaches and TMD (temporomandibular disorder), a jaw problem with a variety of symptoms. (See chapter 2 for more information on TMD.) For some people, incorrectly positioned teeth and jaws can exacerbate speech difficulties and chewing problems; correcting your bite by straightening your teeth can help improve both.

Ask your general dentist about teeth straightening or see a specialist (called an "orthodontist") who performs orthodontics, or teeth straightening. Again—and I can't emphasize it enough—do your research and ask questions so you can decide which option and dentist will work best for you. Perhaps do several consults, with both a general dentist and a specialist. Listen to what each has to say, and choose based on what you hear and your comfort level with the dentist.

It's true that braces aren't just for kids anymore, especially with some of the treatment options available today, including Invisalign®, ClearCorrect™, Six Month Smiles®, and lingual braces. These new types of braces aren't nearly as visible as traditional braces made of ceramic or metal, which are still available, of course, if the other options aren't right for you.

Your best option depends on your current dental situation, your goals, and your budget. Let's discuss clear aligners and Six Month Smiles in depth.

Clear Aligners (Invisalign and ClearCorrect)

Invisalign and ClearCorrect are methods that use nearly invisible, comfortable, clear trays, or aligners, as an alternative to using metal braces to align teeth for both teens and adults. Better yet, these are fast and easy methods. The trays are removable, so you can take them out to eat and clean your teeth. According to the company Align Technology, Inc., which designs, manufactures, and markets clear, removable aligners, nearly 80 percent of all adults are good candidates for using the aligners.

For people who have complex teeth-straightening cases, we refer them to an orthodontic specialist. These clients are typically *not* good candidates for aligners because their teeth need more force to move them than the aligners can apply.

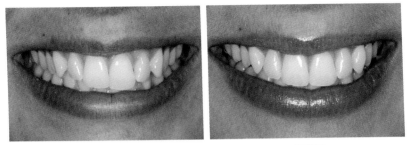

BEFORE   AFTER

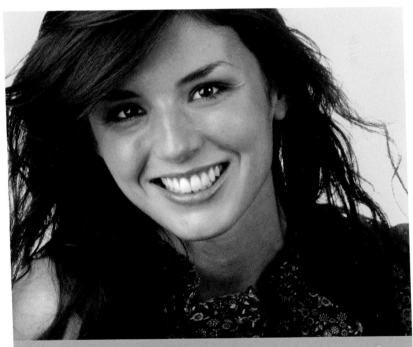

Carson had great teeth shapes and shade; she just wanted to straighten them. She wore Invisalign for just five months.

Main Advantages of Clear Aligners vs. Traditional Braces

- Most people won't notice your teeth are being straightened.
- Treatment won't disrupt your lifestyle.
- Method has no metal wires or bands to irritate your mouth.

We often prescribe straightening treatment alone or with some contouring and whitening, or as an adjunct to veneers, implants, or bridges. Using aligners allows us to set up a person's teeth to obtain the ideal result. If we plan to use aligners as an adjunct to veneers, then the result won't be compromised because teeth are in the ideal positions as opposed to doing veneers without straightening first. As discussed in chapter 2, instant orthodontics involves correcting the smile without braces first, which has some positives and negatives. After all, people will have their veneers for a long time, so it's worth a few months of waiting to get the ideal result. It's often healthier for the teeth, too.

Most frequently, we see clients who have crowded or crooked bottom teeth and want veneers on their top teeth. We then set up aligners to straighten the bottom teeth and move the top teeth to ideal locations for veneers. They may wear the aligners on the top teeth for only a couple of months but may continue to wear aligners on the bottom teeth for a year or more.

The Clear Aligner Procedure Explained

At your first visit, we take photographs, x-rays, and impressions of your teeth. Following our specific directions, the company that makes the trays then uses all of these to make a series of custom aligners for your teeth.

At your second visit, we give you the first three sets of aligners. We attach tooth-colored buttons (made from filling material) to some teeth to help the aligners move your teeth. If your teeth are crowded, a set of sanding strips may be used to create small spaces between your teeth.

Invisalign's Treatment at a Glance

1. An Invisalign-certified orthodontist or dentist evaluates your teeth and creates a program of treatment. At this stage, photos and impressions of your teeth are taken.

2. Align Technology makes a CT scan (computed tomography, or CAT scan) from your dental impressions. The CT scan produces an extremely accurate 3-D digital model of your teeth.

3. CAD (computer-aided design) software is then used to simulate the movement of your teeth during treatment.

4. Your dentist/orthodontist reviews, modifies, and approves the treatment plan before the aligners are created.

5. Align Technology then uses advanced stereolithography (SLA) technology to build precise molds of your teeth at each stage of your treatment.

6. Individualized, custom-created clear aligners are made from these models and sent to your dentist's or orthodontist's office.

7. You wear each aligner for approximately two weeks. Your progress is monitored until you have a wonderful smile.

At subsequent visits, you get your next set of three aligners and we perform any tooth adjustments that need to be made. Typically, we see you every six weeks, each time giving you three new aligners that you change every two weeks. The trays are numbered to help you keep track. Beware that your teeth will be the sorest when you change trays, so we suggest taking an over-the-counter pain reliever such as Ibuprofen to help with your transition from tray to tray.

On average, a client wears these aligners for nine months, but we've known cases to require a range anywhere from three to 18 months. By comparison, regular braces are typically worn for at least two years.

After this treatment, you must wear some type of retainer. Without it, your teeth can shift right back to where they were before treatment. That's why we recommend using some kind of retainer for life. You definitely want to prevent any shifting from taking place.

Cleanings Are Much Easier!

Unlike traditional orthodontics or braces, the aligner technology has no metal bands or wires to trap food and plaque. Maintaining a good oral hygiene program will also reduce chances of plaque buildup, tooth decay, and periodontal disease.

Teeth that are crowded or too widely spaced can create unhealthy conditions, including swollen gums, redness, and pocketing, all of which are signs of periodontal disease. Clinical studies have shown that gum health may improve with the use of aligners during orthodontic treatment. Properly aligned teeth can help gums "fit" tighter around each tooth. This, in turn, may lead to better periodontal health. Unlike with traditional braces, with aligners you can brush and floss normally, which always helps prevent tooth decay and gum disease. (See chapter 9 for details on home care for your teeth.)

Helpful Ways to Use Clear Aligner Technology

Make sure your trays are seating well when you switch them at home. The aligners should slip down all the way over your teeth and snap over the buttons. If your tray doesn't go down, stay in your current tray for another 24 hours, then try again. If you're still having problems, give your dentist a call to help you troubleshoot.

The aligners start out crystal clear, but after seven to 10 days, they start to look cloudy. Make sure you brush them every time you brush your teeth. You can sleep with them in, and you can drink water with them in, but that's it. You should take them out to eat, then brush your teeth before you put your aligners back in your mouth. If you can't brush, then rinse your mouth thoroughly with water. When your aligners look cloudy, you can clean them by brushing and using a denture cleaner to remove the bio film. If that doesn't work, you can put a tablespoon of bleach in a cup of water and allow the aligners to soak for a couple of hours. Rinse and brush the aligners, then enjoy the clean, fresh look.

When you choose this system, you receive two cases: The blue case is for the new aligner, and the red one is for the old. If you lose your aligners, don't panic. Call your dentist immediately and wear the old aligner until your replacement is ordered and received. They aren't cheap, so be careful!

The most uncomfortable time to wear the aligners is when you change to the new set. The new trays make your teeth sorest for the first 24 to 48 hours, so take an over-the-counter painkiller before and after you switch.

It is important to wear your trays at least 22 hours a day. Don't skip days, or you'll prolong treatment. This may lead to complications that make it difficult to get your teeth straight.

Align Technology has established certain requirements making it somewhat difficult for dentists to provide its technology and product. For example, a dentist has to perform a certain number of cases a year and take a certain number of continuing education credits. This is a good thing; it weeds out the dentists who don't use Invisalign very often so the company can concentrate on those who do. But these restrictive requirements also opened the door for other orthodontic companies and their technologies to emerge.

One of them is Six Month Smiles.

Six Month Smiles®

Six Month Smiles provides a modern twist on tried-and-true orthodontics. Braces continue to be the most widely used and most effective way to give patients straight, healthy teeth and a beautiful smile. So Six Month Smiles has taken the best aspects of braces and modified the treatment and materials. Specifically, it uses clear composite brackets in conjunction

Features and Benefits of Six Month Smiles

- Average treatment time is only six months.
- Clear brackets and tooth-colored wires are barely visible.
- The braces are comfortable.
- Safe and effective light forces are used for a shorter time than with conventional braces.
- The cost is typically lower than for traditional braces. Most dentists charge between $2,900 and $6,900 for Six Month Smiles. Many include retainers and teeth whitening as part of a Six Month Smiles package.

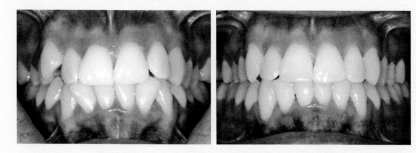

BEFORE   **AFTER**

This patient received Six Month Smiles to correct her crooked teeth and give her a pretty smile. Photos compliments of Dr. Michael Barr.

with Teflon-coated, tooth-colored NiTi (biocompatible nickel titanium) wires. The resulting braces are inconspicuous, which patients greatly appreciate. This option gives them a common-sense, cosmetic solution that fits their lifestyle.

Traditional vs. Short-term Orthodontics

Six Month Smiles is able to tout short treatment times because the goals of treatment differ slightly from those of traditional orthodontics. Traditional orthodontics aim to achieve a finish as close as possible to the "ideal." To do this requires achieving a number of dental objectives.

A short-term orthodontic treatment like Six Months Smile is defined as a treatment that lasts for less than six months and is cosmetically focused. Its goal is to correct the patient's main concerns and create as much symmetry as possible during the treatment time. These goals are consistent with most orthodontic treatment given with clear aligners or those "invisible braces" you may have seen on TV. In this procedure, the way your back teeth come together usually doesn't change significantly, although minor bite discrepancies can be corrected with short-term treatment.

Most adults who are unhappy with their smiles have tooth position problems that can be addressed with a short-term orthodontic treatment. Those who have more serious complaints would probably not be good candidates for this treatment.

Although most orthodontists don't advertise short-term treatments, they do offer some types of "compromised treatment" if a patient declines traditional treatment or jaw surgery. Most treatments using clear aligners offered by orthodontists and general dentists aren't meant to provide an "ideal" result.

We know from experience that a significant amount of tooth movement can be safely accomplished in fewer than six months. However, correcting major dental issues, such as jaw size discrepancy, center lines that don't match up, or a large overjet, usually involves years of treatment for adult patients. For this reason, correction of these problems normally falls outside the scope of short-term orthodontics.

Lingual Braces

Lingual braces provide a way to accomplish major tooth movement without having all the orthodontic hardware on the outsides of the teeth. In this treatment, the braces are on the insides of the teeth, hiding the fact that you're straightening your teeth. Most general dentists don't offer this option, so you'd need to see an orthodontist who performs this procedure frequently.

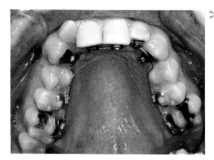

✳ This photo shows lingual braces on the backs of the teeth. These braces cannot be seen from the front when the patient smiles or talks.

You now know various options for straightening your teeth, so you can choose one that best fits your situation. The next chapter explains another aspect of achieving a beautiful smile—bonding and contouring.

*

Chapter 5

Are You a Candidate for Bonding and Contouring?

We have a number of clients who would love to improve their smiles using porcelain veneers, but this option is not in their budgets. For these clients, we start discussing a less expensive option to make improvements to the smile.

Bonding and contouring can also be used on clients who need only minor modifications to their smile. This treatment may or may not be recommended by your dentist, because not all dentists are well trained or comfortable performing this procedure. So when getting consults on ways to improve your smile, you can ask for a less expensive option if porcelain veneers are too much for your budget. Your dentist should be able to explain what changes can be made and show photos of patient outcomes.

Bonding

Dentists have long been using tooth-colored bonding material called composite to repair chipped, cracked, or disfigured front teeth and replace silver amalgam on back teeth. Bonding is appropriate when your goals involve minor changes or your budget is limited. Using bonding techniques, your new smile can often be completed in one visit.

Bonding may also be used to create composite veneers. In this procedure, the dentist improves your smile using composite material to make your veneers in the office directly on your teeth. In contrast, porcelain veneers are made of porcelain and made by a lab.

Porcelain veneers can look more natural, but composite veneers are a less expensive alternative. A small number of dentists are highly skilled at creating composite veneers and can make them look similar to porcelain veneers. However, some dentists can make even porcelain veneers look bad. Again, it's not the treatment, it's the dentist.

Bottom line? Composite veneers are less expensive and can be completed in one visit, if cost and time are of concern. But they may not look as natural as porcelain veneers; they don't last as long in most cases; and typically, major length changes can't be made to the composites.

The procedure involves roughening a tooth's surface, applying the bonding material, and sculpting it into shape, followed

Whiten Teeth First

Do you whiten your teeth before bonding? Yes, most of our clients do the whitening first, then bond to match their lighter-color teeth.

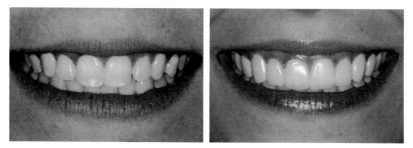

BEFORE   **AFTER**

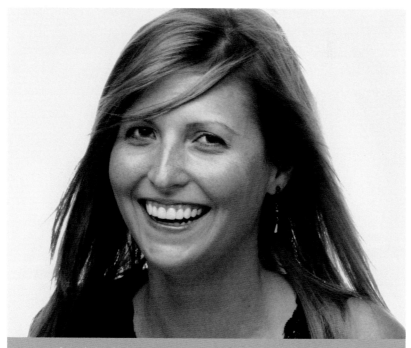

Krystal originally wanted ten porcelain veneers. After discussing her budget, however, we decided to do ten composite veneers to achieve her goals of a bigger and whiter smile.

by hardening the composite with a curing light and polishing the new surface. When enhancing your front teeth in this way, anesthesia is not usually needed.

Bonding can improve the appearance of upper or lower teeth by filling in cavities or imperfections, chips, uneven surfaces, and gaps. It may be a good way to change the size, shape, and position of your teeth, depending on your situation. For slight rotations and small chips, bonding can last seven to 10 years. It's less expensive than porcelain veneers, but when more correction is needed, applying porcelain veneers is a stronger, longer-lasting alternative.

Because bonding isn't as strong as natural front teeth, you have to be careful when biting into hard foods. Opening packages with your teeth and biting your nails can harm your bonding, just as it can damage your natural teeth.

Care of Your Newly Bonded Teeth

Typically, you can eat, drink, brush, and floss as you normally do after having this procedure (later that day). Bonded teeth should receive the same meticulous care as natural teeth. As always, regular brushing, flossing, and tongue scraping as well as professional preventive treatments are necessary to maintain proper oral health and appearance.

To enhance the longevity and maintain the natural appearance of cosmetic bonding, avoid excessive consumption of stain-producing foods, beverages, and tobacco products.

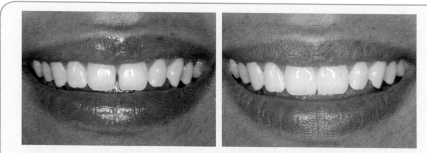

BEFORE   AFTER

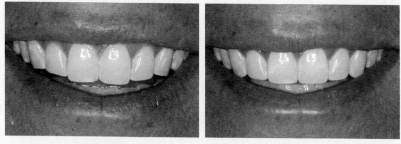

BEFORE   AFTER

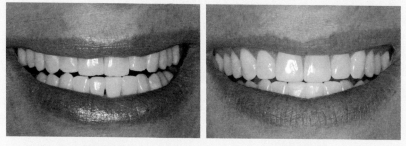

BEFORE   AFTER

These patients all liked their smiles but wanted some minor tweaking, such as closing a space, correcting chips, and reversing an aging smile.

The Pros and Cons of Bonding

Pros

- Bonding is a conservative procedure.
- The procedure is fast, usually taking place in only one visit.
- There is no downtime, and post-op discomfort is minimal.
- Bonding looks natural.
- Bonding is relatively less expensive than more durable cosmetic options.

Cons

- Bonding breaks and stains more easily than porcelain options.
- Highly technique sensitive. The dentist needs to possess an artistic eye and hand.
- Very few dentists have the skill to make bonded teeth look as good as porcelain veneers.

Contouring

Contouring, or shaping the teeth, can be an affordable and painless procedure. Just a few minutes in the dental studio can give your smile a beautiful new look, as painlessly as filing your nails. You'll find a little fine-tuning can go a long way.

A good candidate for contouring has healthy teeth that are uneven in appearance but with a fairly uniform arch. However, grossly uneven teeth may not be as ideal for this procedure. A qualified dentist can help you decide what will work best for you.

In the contouring process, nothing is added to a tooth, only taken away. The dentist removes small areas of your enamel by

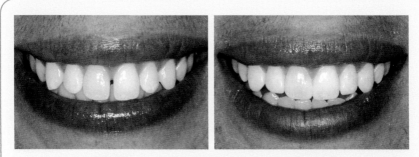

BEFORE   AFTER

Joel wanted to close the gap between his teeth, reduce the sharpness of his canines, and add some length to his laterals to give him a more masculine-looking smile. We used a combination of bonding and contouring to achieve these goals.

sanding and shaping to resolve imperfections—just like an artist working on a sculpture. You'll see that minor reshaping can create the illusion of better alignment or more uniform length.

Rarely does the procedure feel uncomfortable, but if it does, the dentist can use local anesthesia. In our office, we sometimes combine contouring with bonding and a veneer or two to achieve an attractive, even smile. Bonding is typically used in conjunction with contouring to create the proper balance of adding and taking away. This process can result in minor or even major improvements, but it isn't used when big structural changes are necessary. Again, the teeth are often bleached first to the desired color, and then the bonding is added to match that lighter color. Contouring is relatively quick and inexpensive.

Now that we've addressed how your teeth can be improved, let's talk about lifting your gums to further improve your smile in the next chapter.

The Pros and Cons of Contouring

Pros

- Contouring is normally painless.
- The procedure requires only one visit.
- Contouring is inexpensive.

Cons

- Contouring is irreversible.

*

Chapter 6

The Stunning Effects of a Gum Lift

The ideal position for your upper lip when you're smiling is right where your gums meet your front two teeth, or slightly above or below that juncture. If your smile is too "gummy" (meaning too much gum shows when you smile), you can research several techniques to correct it.

Often a combination of two or more procedures is used to obtain optimal results. Your dentist and either a plastic surgeon, an oral surgeon, or a periodontist conduct the surgery. Surgical choices include crown lengthening, lip repositioning, and orthognathic surgery, which are discussed here. Also, Botox is a new way dentists are decreasing the gumminess in gummy smiles.

Crown Lengthening (Traditional and Laser Gum Lift)

Probably the most common method of improving a gummy smile is a procedure that removes and contours the gum tissue. Some of the gum tissue is removed above the tooth, making the teeth longer. This change in the ratio of "pink" (gums) to "white" (teeth) makes a big difference in the overall appearance of a smile.

Crown lengthening is ideal when excess gum tissue covers teeth, making them look too short. Once the gum tissue is removed, the teeth appear normal in length. In some cases, root tissue gets exposed, so porcelain veneers or bonding can then be used to aesthetically enhance the teeth and cover the exposed root surfaces. Some patients have normal tooth length already, so lifting the gums would make the teeth appear too long. In this case, they're referred to a specialist to learn more about one of the other treatments available.

Some of our clients initially "freak out" about this crown-lengthening procedure. But we assure them it's relatively fast and easy, and they tolerate it well and heal quickly (as I did). If only a small amount of gum tissue is removed, healing can occur within 24 to 48 hours. If some of the bone around the teeth has to be removed, full recovery may take about 10 to 14 days. The procedure, which can be completed in one appointment, takes anywhere from five minutes to one hour and can be done under local anesthesia. Laser gum lifts are fairly quick, easy, and inexpensive, producing predictable results with minimal recovery time.

We like the accuracy and fast healing that lasers provide, but they're expensive, so a large number of dentists still perform gum lifts the traditional way. With the traditional procedure, the patient is numbed and the gums are partially removed with a scalpel; they are then peeled back so bone can be removed. Finally, the gums are sutured back into place. Negatives of this traditional method include longer healing time (four to six weeks) and a painful recovery. With both methods, sometimes a touch up is needed after the gums heal.

We use the laser to contour tissue on a large number of our smile makeover clients. Rarely are someone's gum heights perfect on every tooth. This procedure helps balance out the gums and teeth to obtain greater symmetry while adding that extra touch to a natural-looking, gorgeous smile. It can be performed on eight to 10 teeth, or just on one tooth that's too short. This minor change results in more balance in a smile that may have otherwise looked "off."

Post-procedure Instructions for Laser Gum Lifts

- For two days following the procedure, use the clear syringe with hydrogen peroxide three times a day to rinse your mouth and gums and kill bacteria.
- Use the rubber tip stimulator twice a day for four days to push gently into the gums, like pushing back your cuticle on your fingernail. This prevents the fibers from reattaching.
- Don't brush the area where the teeth were treated for 12 hours. On the evening following your procedure, you can start brushing very gently with a soft toothbrush.
- Stay on a soft-food diet of mostly fish and pasta to avoid biting with your front teeth for one to two days.
- Take 800 mg of Motrin the night before and the morning of your procedure, and again after your procedure, typically before the numbness wears off.

Two types of lasers are used by dentists to contour gum tissue. A diode laser is used only on soft gum tissue for minor corrections of tissue height when enhancing a smile. It's a reasonably affordable laser for dentists, so it's becoming more common. The other type of laser is an Er:YAG (Erbium YAG). The Er:YAG laser can contour soft tissue like the gums and also contour the bone underneath the gums. This capability is important if less subtle changes need to be made in tooth lengths.

Using the Er:YAG laser, first the gums are partially removed, making the tooth the ideal length for the smile. Then the settings are changed on the laser, and the bone is contoured to an ideal distance from the new gum height. Although fewer dentists own an Er:YAG than a diode laser because of the expense, it's an extremely valuable tool in a cosmetic dentist's arsenal because it allows full control of the gum heights. The majority of our smile makeovers are enhanced by the careful manipulation of gum heights utilizing both our diode and Er:YAG lasers.

Lip Repositioning

Typically performed by a plastic surgeon or periodontist, a simple lip-repositioning procedure can have dramatic results. Our practice doesn't perform this surgery, so I mention it not from personal experience but as an option. You will need to research the right professional to perform it. Although most often used in conjunction with crown lengthening, lip positioning can be effective in itself.

Just the words—lip repositioning—sound drastic, don't they? But the procedure is not. It involves removing a small portion of the tissue on the inside of your upper lip and suturing the lip to the gums. The procedure doesn't change the

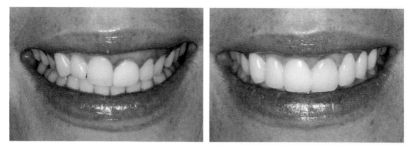

BEFORE   AFTER

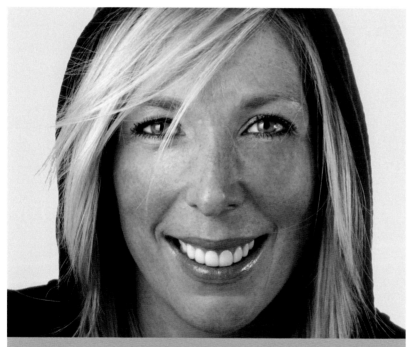

Aine received a laser gum lift and eight veneers to achieve her goals of a less gummy smile and bigger and whiter teeth.

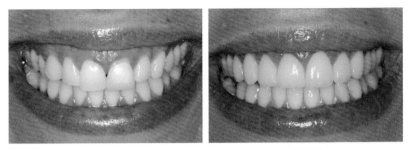

BEFORE   AFTER

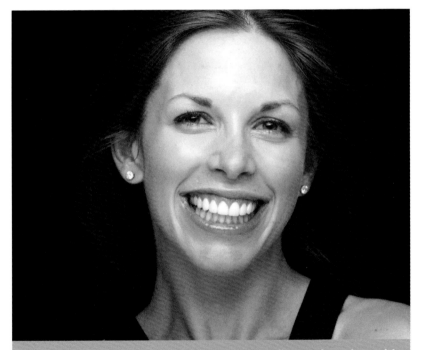

Shylo wanted to reduce her gummy smile, replace her old crown, and have a whiter smile, so we did a laser gum lift, one crown, and seven veneers.

appearance of your face. Rather, it prevents the muscles in your lip from raising your lip too high when you smile and showing too much gum tissue. It's capable of achieving optimal results if the lip needs to be repositioned 10 mm or fewer. Typically done under local anesthesia, the procedure lasts about one hour. Patients usually experience some swelling, particularly during the first few days, but it's barely noticeable after one week and completely gone in two weeks.

Lip repositioning is considered a fairly fast, easy, and inexpensive way to achieve dramatic results with a quick recovery.

Botox

Botox, typically used to reduce wrinkles, is now being used to weaken or relax the muscles pulling up on the lip, resulting in a reduction in gum display of the smile. This treatment may be used by itself or in combination with gum contouring. Different amounts of Botox are used to reduce the gum display by 3 to 6 mm. Pros of Botox are that it is conservative and cost effective, and the effects wear off in three to four months in case you don't like it. On the negative side, it doesn't last, and as the results wear off, you need to get more Botox.

Orthognathic Surgery

More extensive than the other two lip-repositioning procedures, orthognathic surgery involves moving the jawbones. Most often this surgery is used to move the upper jaw and correct a gummy smile or to move the lower jaw forward or backward to correct a person's profile. Before the surgery, patients generally have orthodontic treatment to position their teeth as ideally as possible.

Orthognathic surgery can take anywhere from a few hours to as many as eight hours. Once the surgery is completed, braces are installed to wire the mouth closed for about one month while the bone fuses. Healing can take as long as several months in severe cases.

The downside of this procedure can be daunting. In addition to its expense, your jaws need to be wired shut after surgery. The procedure requires a difficult and lengthy recovery. In addition, you might experience residual numbness in the affected parts of your mouth and chin that could last months—or the rest of your life.

As with any cosmetic procedure, do your research, ask a lot of questions, and examine photos of the professionals' work before you decide which option is right for you.

As you focus on a creating better, healthier smile for all to see, don't forget about the back part of your mouth, which is addressed in the next chapter.

Chapter 7
Natural-Look Fillings of Back-Tooth Dentistry

Cosmetic enhancements are not just for your front teeth; your back teeth can benefit from cosmetics as well. Back-tooth restorations include fillings, inlays and onlays, crowns, bridges, and implants.

Most people are aware of cavities or dental decay and the need to take care of these problems before they lose their teeth. Unfortunately, cavities don't heal on their own; they need to be repaired and/or restored. Fillings today are most commonly made of a plastic material called composite or porcelain. In most cosmetic dental offices, these tooth-colored materials have replaced the mercury-containing, silver-colored amalgam fillings; however, both gold and amalgam are still widely used in family-style or insurance-driven practices.

Amalgam has been the material of choice for more than 100 years, but over the years, people have debated the health risks of amalgam fillings. Yes, amalgam contains mercury, but when it's combined with metals such as silver, copper, and tin, it forms a stable alloy. The Food and Drug Administration (FDA) has studied amalgam and declared it to be safe. However, numerous studies contradict the FDA's position.

What do I think? I don't necessarily believe everything I've read about the negative effects of mercury, but I did have my silver fillings replaced. I also have a mercury-free office and wouldn't use it for my young son's fillings. Some states require offices to have a specific trap in the dental lines to prevent the mercury from contaminating the environment. That implies it's bad for the environment; is it not also bad for my body? Hmmm. I say, better safe than sorry. Replace those silver fillings and insist on non-amalgam fillings in the future. There may be very few specific cases when a composite filling may be too difficult to isolate and place, so perhaps an amalgam filling would be best. An educated, experienced dentist will know when and why the benefits would outweigh the risks.

Definition of Terms

filling—the result of filling a cavity, or hole, in a tooth with composite or porcelain, gold, or silver amalgam

inlays and onlays—types of restoration used to restore a tooth when a filling isn't enough yet a crown is too much

crown—a restoration that covers the entire tooth, restoring the tooth's anatomy, function, and aesthetics

bridge—a restoration to replace one or more missing teeth that uses teeth adjacent to the missing tooth/teeth as anchors

implant—a metal fixture inserted in the bone that serves as the root or base for an artificial tooth when one or more teeth are missing

Another negative characteristic is that amalgam expands as it sets, and continues to expand, so it may eventually cause a tooth to crack or break, especially with large silver fillings. Also, amalgam fillings remain in your mouth long after they start to leak and cause problems for the tooth. Therefore, make sure your dentist checks your old amalgams frequently. Because amalgams show up bright white on a radiograph, cavities can form under them and often go undiagnosed by a dentist for a long time. For this reason, we recommend taking out older amalgams that look as if they no longer form a good seal in the tooth.

I do see why some dentists might oppose the newer composite fillings because of insurance, cost, or the fact that they're difficult to place. The procedure is quite technique sensitive, and if not done well, the filling doesn't last very long. However, composite or porcelain fillings are believed to strengthen the tooth, not weaken it. So ask your own dentist about his or her beliefs and recommendations. If you question the answers you receive, seek other dentists to consult.

The bottom line is that, in the past, the only options for fillings were silver and gold. Even though these options are still available, most common today are composite and porcelain fillings, which are explained here.

Composite/Resin Fillings: This tooth-colored material can provide a highly natural look if the dentist has patience and does it right. The procedure normally includes anesthetizing the area and drilling out the cavity or the existing filling to be replaced. Then the composite is placed in the tooth in small increments. A light (UV or laser) is used to harden, or cure, the material, and then the filling is adjusted using the drill and bite paper to make it fit properly with your bite. Finally, the new composite is polished. *Important:* This procedure should be done using either a rubber dental dam or a device such as Isolite that allows the area to remain dry. Why? Because allowing the tooth or filling to become contaminated with saliva is a common reason these fillings fail. Also, if you're having silver filings removed, these two methods—along with a high-speed suction device—help suction up the mercury vapors.

Porcelain Inlays and Onlays: Using porcelain restoration to fill a tooth is similar to installing a partial crown; it can look extremely natural and virtually invisible if done well. "Inlay" means the restoration is within the tooth; "onlay" means the restoration wraps over some or all of the cusps. Inlays are used when tooth structure can sufficiently hold the filling, while onlays are used when part of the tooth is compromised and can't hold all the filling. Crowns are also used for this reason.

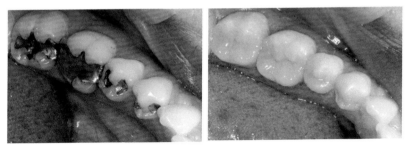

BEFORE   AFTER

Onlays cover part of the tooth's surface, while crowns cover the entire tooth. However, applying crowns is usually a more aggressive procedure because more tooth structure needs to be drilled away. Again, which one is used depends on the education and experience of the dentist. In our office, we use the most conservative treatment and don't do many crowns anymore unless we're replacing old ones.

Inlays, onlays, and crowns may also be made out of gold. Gold lasts a long time and rarely breaks. The downside? Gold teeth can make you look like a pirate—not a cosmetically pleasing look! Also, gold is softer than enamel and can wear thin over time if a person has an incorrect bite. Most patients won't realize it's getting thinner until the tooth underneath begins to show. Someone with a stable bite, however, would find that gold is quite durable.

Porcelain inlays, onlays, and crowns can be made in two ways. Most commonly, a lab fabricates the restoration, which requires you to wear a temporary restoration for two to three weeks while the permanent piece is being made. This also requires a second visit to remove the temporary and to cement on the permanent restoration. Another method features new technology that allows you to leave the dentist's chair sporting your restoration the same day. Names for this type of fabrication include CAD/CAM, CEREC, and E4D. It's fast because a machine mills your permanent restoration right in the office while you're waiting.

As with everything, each approach has pros and cons. In our office, we don't own a CAD/CAM machine because we think the restorations from our lab look more natural (as discussed in chapter 8). Some dentists may love this new technology and take their time to make the results look great. But I wouldn't use CAD/CAM restorations for front teeth or smile makeovers because of the esthetics *and* because patients don't get to test-drive their new smiles (shades and shapes) first.

Another complaint we've heard about CAD/CAM restorations is they're not as smooth and polished as some of the other work people have received in the past. Again, I believe this comes down to the dentist, not necessarily the technology. So interview your dentist and other dentists thoroughly to see what's best for you and your mouth. Know that the appearance of your back teeth can be improved with a composite filling, veneer, inlay, onlay, or crown, depending on what they need and the level of skill the dentist has achieved to deliver it.

Crowns: Why might one of your teeth need a crown? It could be broken or cracked or may have undergone a root canal. A crown becomes like a false tooth. The most common materials to construct crowns are ceramic and porcelain fused to metal (PFM). PFM crowns use metal as the substructure, which results in showing a "black" line around the gum line. Because of more cosmetic options available, we haven't placed a PFM in nearly five years in our office. However, PFMs are less expensive than ceramic, so if you don't care about the aesthetic aspects, they may be a good option for you.

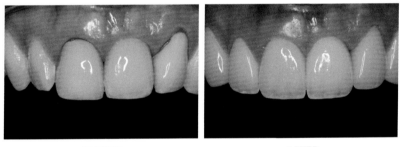

BEFORE   AFTER

If you care what your crown looks like, consider an all-ceramic crown. Many choices of ceramic are available; consult with your dentist to decide which is best for you. Factors determining choices include color of the tooth, how much of the tooth is left, the forces endured by this area of the mouth, and how it will look. After conferring with your dentist, you might select a CAD/CAM crown. Be sure to ask about the pros and cons and, most important, inquire about the dentist's experience with this technique. You want to feel comfortable about your choice.

> # New Option Available
>
> A word on IPS e.max, which is all the buzz now: IPS e.max is a type of porcelain made of lithium disilicate that's twice as strong as traditional porcelains. It has even more fracture strength than crowns that are reinforced with metal and zirconium. Look for this option to become more popular.

Bridges: Bridge structures provide a way to replace a missing tooth either in the front or the back of the mouth. Many different types of bridges are available, and each one is best used in certain circumstances.

Here's how a bridge is constructed: The dentist places a crown on the tooth in front of the space where the tooth is missing, a crown on the tooth behind the space, and a fake tooth in the middle; then all three are connected with a three-unit bridge. A bridge can replace a number of teeth and involve additional anchor teeth.

Sometimes a bridge is constructed with only one anchor tooth supporting the fake tooth (instead of anchor teeth on either side of the fake tooth) and involving only two units (instead of three or more). Called a "cantilever bridge," it's used only under certain circumstances. (I have two cantilever bridges replacing my laterals, which were missing for genetic reasons.) Like crowns, bridges can be made of metal, porcelain and metal, or all porcelain, and can be constructed in a lab or using a CAD/CAM machine.

A more conservative bridge option is called a "Maryland" bridge. This type of bridge doesn't crown the adjacent teeth; rather, it uses wings on the backs of those teeth to hold the fake tooth. It's a great option for the front teeth, but sometimes not strong enough for back teeth.

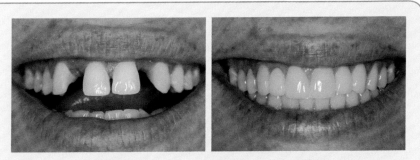

BEFORE   AFTER

This patient wanted to replace her genetically missing teeth with a natural-looking treatment, as well as whiten her teeth and correct the premature wear. *Full disclosure:* This is me! This was what my teeth looked like before Jason restored my smile with two bridges, two crowns, and sixteen veneers. Thanks, honey!

Dental Implants: Another approach to replacing missing teeth is the use of dental implants. The implant serves as the root of the tooth, and a crown goes on top to take the place of the missing tooth. Three separate pieces are involved: (1) the actual implant in the bone, (2) the abutment, which screws into the implant and sticks through the gums, and (3) the crown, which is either cemented or screwed on the abutment. The implant is surgically inserted into the jawbone. Usually, it's left alone to heal and integrate for four to six months, although sometimes a temporary crown can be placed on an implant right away. In some cases, there's not adequate bone available for the implant, so some type of graft must be done first. In other cases, the bone quality and quantity are excellent and the crown may be placed immediately.

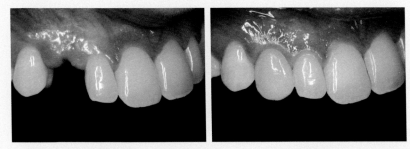

BEFORE   **AFTER**

Kelsey was born without her canine tooth, so we decided to use an implant here instead of a flipper (not permanent) or a bridge (too aggressive). Our goals were for her gums, as well as the crown on top of the implant, to look great.

Numerous types of implants abound, and the technology keeps changing rapidly. That's why it's important to do your research. General dentists, as well as specialists like perio-dontists and oral surgeons, can place implants. Implants can also help retain loose dentures or non-removable bridges that replace an entire arch of missing teeth. *Bonus:* Implants decrease or prevent bone loss. When teeth are missing, the bone tends to shrink or disappear, which can be disastrous for denture wear-ers. This bone loss may also compromise the cosmetics of a smile because the bone in that area appears sunken.

All the techniques discussed here lead to what's addressed in the next chapter—how to choose the best dentist for your beautiful smile.

＊

Chapter 8

How to Research and Choose Your Smile Makeover Dentist

Now that you have a thorough understanding of cosmetic dentistry procedures, it's time to consider the most important decision of all—choosing your dentist.

Warning. You are making a permanent change to your face—do your research!

As I mentioned in the introduction to this book, I've noticed what seems to be a widespread complacency—or maybe it's ignorance—among dentists that results in less-than-ideal smile designs. I see photographs of subpar results in many of the cosmetic dentistry trade publications. Thousands of dentists read these magazines for educational purposes, so when they see less-than-high-quality work validated, they continue to make mediocre smiles.

However, certain dentists have obtained a different kind of education more geared to understanding the principles of smile design. These dentists are well versed in the materials and techniques involved. They've spent far more time and money on smile makeover education than general dentists have.

Unfortunately, in most states they aren't allowed to advertise to make the public more aware of their knowledge any more than a complacent dentist who creates subpar smiles can. This hurts the public. That's why it's up to you, the consumer, to do your research.

Advertising rules differ from state to state; many states regulate what can and cannot be said in a dentist's advertising. In Florida, for example, we can't state anything that's laudatory, meaning anything that makes us sound better than other dentists. Nor can we claim to be experts in cosmetics or state that it's our specialty. In fact, in 2006 when we first opened our new studio, we were fined $4,000 because our ads said "advanced dentistry" and one published interview called Jason

Genesis of Problem

Here's the basic problem as I see it: The term "cosmetic dentist" means absolutely nothing, and there are no regulations about which dentists can or cannot use this term. This means any dentist can say he or she is a cosmetic dentist; there are no restrictions about it. What happens? Many dentists take advantage of this lack of a legal definition and claim to be cosmetic dentists. They may be somewhat innocent in their claim, thinking they learned enough in dental school or by reading dental magazines. Some feel entirely capable of meeting their patients' desires. However, cosmetic dentistry requires extensive training and a huge commitment of time, money, and energy. So if dentists can use the label "cosmetic dentist" without jumping through educational hoops, what's more expedient for them?

a "perfectionist." (Another dentist in Jacksonville had anonymously turned us in.)

We were also fined for stating we were "state of the art." How many other dentists are making those claims? But unless someone reports inappropriate advertising and a dentist gets fined, many risk saying exactly what they want to say in their advertisements.

Dispelling the Myths and Concerns

In my research, I heard some unbelievable myths from patients, things they said their dentist told them. Let me dismiss a few of them so you'll be more informed as you conduct your research and talk with dentists.

One day, a woman came into our studio for an in-office whitening treatment. She told us her dentist uses only whitening trays because the UV light other dentists use for in-office treatment damages the integrity of the teeth. This is ridiculous. The UV light for this procedure does no such thing. But how many patients now fear improving their smile with this effective process because this dentist with little training in cosmetics claims it's damaging?

This same dental practice also claims that veneers pop off in two years—and so they grind their patients' teeth down and do crowns. Veneers do not pop off in two years, if properly done. It's even more disturbing that this particular practice includes "Cosmetic Dentistry" in its name! So what do you think people assume they do? Of course—cosmetics. How do you think patients feel when their teeth are ground down to spikes and they're given ugly smiles? That's why I cannot stress enough the importance of doing research before choosing a smile makeover dentist. Those people didn't know they needed to research the dentist before proceeding. Now you will!

I suggest getting several consultations and bringing along questions to ask. Only when you're satisfied and you feel confident and comfortable in your choice of dentist should you proceed.

I've listed 10 things to look for when choosing a smile makeover dentist. To stress their importance, I've repeated some points in a few of the sections. I'd rather you read something twice than have you not heed something that could make or break your experience.

Ten Crucial Considerations When Researching a Dentist

1. Training and Experience Are Paramount

Inquire about the dentist's expertise. Make sure your practitioner has advanced postgraduate training with live patients, specifically in the procedures that interest you. There's no substitute for intense hands-on training. He or she should also attend 25 to 65 hours a year of continuing education in cosmetic dentistry. The American Dental Association states that dentists in Florida must take a *minimum* of 25 hours of continuing education each year to maintain their license to practice dentistry. Find dentists who do more than squeak by on their credentials.

Dentists who take pride in staying on top of their game aren't shy about telling you where and how much they've

The Importance of Advanced Education in Cosmetic Dentistry

The ability to create knockout smiles should not be taken lightly. Most dentists graduate from dental school with little to no knowledge about smile makeovers. It's up to the dentist to take the state-of-the-art postgraduate training that's available. What training do the dentists you're researching have in smile design? Don't be afraid to ask! A live-patient, hands-on course is a must—and not one they took a decade ago. Dentists need to attend every few years to keep up with the advancements and new techniques.

trained. Never hesitate to ask. Trust me, if the dentist loves this type of work, he or she will love to share postgraduate education accomplishments with you. Look online for a dentist's training credentials. Often, the best dentists not only attend classes, forums, and lectures, but also are hired to instruct other dentists.

2. Latest Technology Matters

Find a progressive practice. Dentists using the latest high-tech equipment and materials are more likely to be up to date on the most recent treatments. For example, the use of diagnostic computers, intra-oral cameras, lasers, and digital x-rays indicates a leading-edge practice. Do they have a computer anesthetic delivery system (a computer that administers the anesthetic slowly and safely) and a T-scan (a computer that checks occlusion, which is the way teeth come together when a person bites)? Finding out about their equipment factors strongly when qualifying various dentists.

3. Extensive Consultation First

Demand quality face time. You have the right to a thorough consultation with the dentist who will be doing your work. If the procedures involve smile makeovers, you should have an opportunity to spend up to an hour, to sit down and describe what you want, ask questions, and go over the procedures, costs, and expectations. An honorable clinician will be up front with you about everything.

A Word on Laboratories

Dental laboratories employ ceramists to make veneers and crowns. Ceramists are artists who create lifelike tooth restorations out of porcelain that's less than half a millimeter thick—about half as thick as your fingernail. They need to be able to create beautiful smiles by understanding the fundamentals of smile design and the way your teeth come together. It's no surprise that the best ceramists in the country make an extremely good living at what they do and are in high demand by excellent dentists. Our studio has the privilege of working with the talented ceramists at Gold Dust Dental Lab in Tempe, Arizona. These ceramists have styled the teeth of superstars and models, and they do the ceramics for some of the best dentists in the country.

Beware of dentists who use inexpensive labs to do veneers. It's not a good way to save money in the process of creating your new smile. Typically, the results are less than ideal and the teeth look artificial. This anecdote will raise your eyebrows: One of these corner-cutting dentists who uses a cheap lab for his patients asked us what lab we use. He was making over his father's smile and wanted to use a "good" lab for this situation. Oh! Your paying patients aren't good enough for the better lab? How sad!

Yes, veneers cost more money when done correctly with quality material, but keep in mind, you will be living with the results for a long time.

Find a professional who will truly listen to your hopes and desires. Despite their relatively low numbers, you can find well-trained, excellent cosmetic dentists all over the country. You deserve someone who will give you personalized care and customized treatment.

4. Laboratory of the Highest Quality

Examine the dentist's lab. Visit the lab's website and look through its portfolios. A dentist should be excited about the materials the practice uses and happy to tell you the name of the lab and the ceramist who produces them. You want these materials to be natural-looking and long-lasting, to provide a beautiful smile that endures. The ceramist will be the other person besides your dentist who will make and design your new look.

5. Cost-Cutting Won't Cut It!

Don't skimp on your smile. Cosmetic dentistry isn't just for celebrities and supermodels anymore. It's surprisingly accessible. Financing plans are available, so don't automatically go for the lowest bidder. Lowballers aren't doing you any favors; they're cutting corners on the quality of materials, or worse, on things that can affect your safety and outcome. If someone offers to do a procedure at far below industry-average prices, be suspicious . . . very suspicious.

6. Member of American Academy of Cosmetic Dentistry (AACD)

Is the dentist a member of the AACD? Ideally, your dentist should be accredited by or working toward accreditation through the American Academy of Cosmetic Dentistry.

Justification of Fees

You'll find a wide range in fees for cosmetic dentistry procedures—similar to the range in talent and education for cosmetic dentists. Prices vary based on

- location in the country and/or area of the city involved,
- increased lab bills for more talented ceramists,
- higher overheads from ongoing costs of education,
- the use of expensive equipment and materials, and
- more individual attention with the doctor, including the likelihood that you will be the only client in the office during your appointment times.

If you choose a dentist based on price alone, I encourage you to find the best one your budget allows. Otherwise, wait until you can accumulate the money to do a smile makeover in a quality manner.

Accreditation requires written and oral exams, submission of clinical case studies, and dedication to continuing education and protocols. Accreditation confers a much higher standard for cosmetic dentistry than the average standard for dentistry. For example, of the 130,000 dentists in the United States, approximately 7,000 of them are members of the AACD, but only about 250 of them are fully accredited.

Keep in mind that there's a big difference between being a member of the organization and being actively involved. I know of many dentists who are members just so they can claim membership on their websites. That doesn't mean anything if they don't attend the meetings or participate.

To learn more, the AACD website provides membership levels for all members, indicating their levels of involvement. Checking this list is an effective way to start your research and begin sorting. That said, I know of several phenomenal dentists who don't participate with the AACD accreditation process (it's just not important to them). This doesn't mean you shouldn't see them for your smile makeover. Just consider using accreditation as another aspect of qualifying a dentist. Be sure to research all areas, not just one or two.

7. Artistic Excellence in Designing Smiles

Pore through photo portfolios of patients or online smile galleries to select an artist who appreciates the nuances that make each smile unique—someone who has the exceptional skills to custom tailor your look. "Smile design" is what those in the industry call the unique art of transforming problem teeth into

Look for Smiles That Appear Natural

Your dentist should consider factors such as mouth shape, bite configuration, size and health of teeth and gum line, color of teeth, your face's shape and skin tone, and much more. But when you look at before-and-after photos of smile design clients, you do not need to think about all the technicalities. Simply look for smiles that appear natural, as they were meant to be. Can you see how the new smile transforms a person's face? You'll find yourself automatically drawn to the smiles that appeal most to you.

It's a good sign if a dentist's office includes a photography studio. Be sure any before-and-after photographs displayed represent the dentist's own patients. Images in portfolios and web galleries should highlight actual cases they've completed. This is critical. Dentists can purchase before-and-after photos of smiles not performed by them. Don't be embarrassed to ask for photos of smiles they've done themselves. And better yet, is there a team member or patient whose smile you can see in real life?

a flawless smile. An inspired cosmetic dentist looks at each smile as a potential work of art, each with its unique challenges and distinctive characteristics.

8. Understanding the Time Involved

Some variations are necessary, but after the initial hour of consultation, most smile makeover procedures require a few more visits of two or more hours, about three weeks apart. A comprehensive pre-op visit should come first to obtain records. The second visit involves all the prep procedures. That's when you'll be fitted for temporary veneers. Then the dentist goes to work with the lab to create the permanent, custom veneers. At your third visit, your new veneers will be cemented into place. A post-op visit may be needed for final adjustments and photos. You shouldn't need any downtime for recovery; most people usually return to their regular routine immediately.

The main point is that the dentist shouldn't be double and triple booked, thus leaving you to sit in the chair waiting or having the assistant do the work. Expect the dentist to work fairly uninterrupted. It's fair to ask about how patients are scheduled and how you would fit in. Use your judgment from the start; if you feel rushed or unimportant during your consultation, then maybe it's not the right place for you. After all, you want a dentist and team who take the time to listen to what you want, and then deliver just that.

9. Form and Function

Of course, you're looking for someone who appreciates the color, luminosity, and shape of a natural-looking smile. The perfect smile marries beauty with durability and functionality. Get honest answers from your dentists regarding how this treatment will affect your bite, your gums, and the general action of your teeth. Ask how long your ceramics should last, what you should do to maintain them, and what you should avoid doing.

Ideally, you'll feel comfortable enough to form a long-term relationship with your smile makeover dentist. That way, should anything go wrong—cracking or chipping—you'll be assured that you'll receive repairs quickly and benefit from ongoing service.

10. Caring Comfort is Key

Going to the dentist is not high on everyone's "love to do" list, but you can expect your dentist to make the experience as comfortable for you as possible—and perhaps you can even expect to be pampered a bit. As you interview dentists, listen to your gut feelings before making a selection. Decide what "little things" are most important to you regarding your dental visit. Validated parking? A soothing atmosphere? Friendly staff? TV and movies for your enjoyment? Find an office that caters to your needs—even spoils you! You should expect to be given star treatment complete with care and discretion.

Side Note

Something to be aware of is marketing and PR. Many dentists spend a tremendous amount of money to be known and heard. We definitely fall in this category; of course we want the people in our community to be aware of who we are and what we do. However, the thing that is so confusing for the consumer is that any dentist can pay for big ads and press; it doesn't necessarily mean he or she is the best dentist in the area. Go ahead and have this dentist on your list to visit, and again, use the above information to research the well-known dentist. Make sure that he or she has the education and passion to back it up and that it's not just all smoke and mirrors.

Beware of Techniques That Are Heavily Marketed

Before you visit the dentists on your list, it's good to be informed about some prepless techniques and products that are marketed heavily and about same-day smile makeovers, two of the most popular innovations in cosmetic dentistry. Both have changed the way many dentists practice, and both have their place in certain situations, but not in all. Let me explain.

Prepless Veneers

This popular technique uses prepless veneers, a form of veneers made from porcelain. The company that makes them does a terrific job at marketing their product, but I believe it misleads the public. Its ads declare that no tooth structure needs to be removed, but if you read the fine print, it states that 0.5 mm may need to be removed—the amount typical for veneer preparation in most cases.

Its ads also state that the process is reversible; you could have these veneers removed if you didn't like them, but only if you have a dentist who is knowledgeable and has the technology to remove them safely. I understand the appeal of that reasoning, but the best insurance isn't whether or not you could have them removed afterward but choosing the right cosmetic dentist in the first place. I've seen patients who had these prepless veneers removed because they hated how bulky their teeth looked. The teeth underneath were scratched and dull looking. It's possible to have them removed safely with a laser and then polished, but again, you need the right dentist to do that for you.

Top cosmetic dentists agree that only a small percentage of cases are good candidates for "no-prep" veneers. "No-prep" means that no tooth structure needs to be removed before placing the veneers—a conservative type of veneer that's becoming more popular. Dr. David Hornbrook and Dr. Dennis Wells, pioneers in cosmetic dentistry, teach the latest techniques in no-prep veneers. But the best dentists do not use the popular marketed prepless veneers. They use their own lab to make these ultra-thin veneers; for example, ours are called Emprethins, and there are other good options available from qualified dentists.

Commercial no-prep veneers are made in a cookie-cutter fashion, which contributes to their artificial and bulky look. Offering no-prep or minimal-prep veneers works if the dentist uses a top-notch lab to handcraft each one, so they look natural. Again, some dentists and patients may love the look of the popular commercial brand. That's fine, as long as people who want a natural look know that no-prep veneers may not be able to give it to them.

If a dentist heavily promotes this type of prepless veneers, then beware. A skilled cosmetic dentist who works with a talented ceramist is likely to think these commercial veneers look bulky, fake, monochromatic, and nonvital compared to a well-done veneer by a preferred ceramist. The country's best ceramists do not work for this popular prepless company; they tend to work at smaller boutique labs that focus on turning out high-quality ceramics.

In my opinion, the no-prep concept is fine; it's the actual product that some patients find fake and bulky looking. By using them, many dentists are compromising the aesthetics of their patients' smiles.

So always examine before-and-after photos of all the types of veneers the dentist offers, and make sure the photos represent his or her actual work. Keep in mind that a heavily marketed no-prep company has a book of before-and-after photos that is given to a dentist who participates in its program. Dentists may be using this brand of veneer because it's relatively inexpensive to learn and implement. We, on the other hand, love to brag about our work and share stories about the patients we show you because we have great confidence in our process and materials. The point here is that even though a product has a well-known name, it may not be right for you, so I still recommend you do your research.

In-office Milled Devices and Materials (One-Day Smile Makeovers)

There are several companies boasting one-day smile makeovers in a process aided by computer technologies such as 3D photography and CAD/CAM. This sounds exciting and may be great for back teeth, where looks aren't critical, but be careful. These same-day crowns and veneers typically don't look or feel as natural as porcelain. A computer is not as artistic as a talented ceramist!

Also, because you get your new veneers in one day, you can't test-drive your smile to be sure you love the color and shapes on your face. Same-day smile makeovers could potentially be a big compromise, so look at many "after" photos up close to be sure the quality is acceptable to you. That said, very few dentists may have mastered this treatment—those who have an artistic eye for what looks good and spend the time to make the milled restorations look natural. But I guarantee that not every dentist using this new technology can tout awesome results. Again, do your research!

Preparing for Your Consultation

Consider your answers to these questions before you consult with a dentist:

- What do you want your smile to be like in five years? 10 years?
- What have you tried already? How did it work?
- How would you rate your smile now, from 1 (embarrassing) to 10 (fabulous)?
- What would it take to make you a perfect 10?
- Have you considered your budget? What is it?

Know your long-term plans and hopes for your teeth and smile. Just taking care of your teeth doesn't necessarily equate to having a beautiful smile. But certainly it's possible to have both healthy teeth and a gorgeous smile. It's up to you what you want for your mouth.

Is there a particular celebrity or movie star whose smile you admire? What aspects of that person's smile draw you to it? It's important for you to know what you consider to be good characteristics, because some of those can be incorporated into your new smile design. Specifically, what would you like to change or improve about your smile? Getting a whiter and straighter smile are the most common requests. Others include replacing missing teeth, making a smile more symmetrical, closing spaces or gaps, lengthening short or worn teeth, making a smile look fuller or wider, younger or older, more feminine or masculine. Some people simply want to replace "old" dentistry.

Lastly, what's your budget? Buying a new smile can cost as much as buying a car. How would you normally pay for a purchase like that? Would you finance it into more manageable payments? If so, you'll need to ask each dentist you interview if this is an option.

Ultimately, you have to determine your goals and set your budget. Often, you can whiten your teeth for the price of a new purse or shoes. You may wear these accessories a few times, but you'll wear your new smile every day. The same goes for a car; you drive it from point A to point B, and some people may notice your fancy wheels, but when you get out of the car, it's your smile that everyone sees for the rest of the day. Do you want a better-looking smile or an absolutely dynamite smile? A pleasant smile or one that dramatically changes your life? All in all, how much is a smile makeover worth to you?

In your consultations, take the opportunity to discuss your goals with the dentists you've selected and find out what type of service they recommend, given your aspirations and budget. Ask many questions, and expect to receive as much time and information as you need. Request to see procedural pictures showing the process of a smile makeover. (Some people like to see *everything*, and some don't. It's up to you.)

Make sure you get as much out of the consult as you can. If you have more questions afterward, or perhaps a spouse or friend raised some concerns, give the dentists you interviewed a call. Their main goal should be to help you make an informed decision. And don't hesitate to ask for additional consultations if you think it would help in your decision making.

After hearing all that, do you get my point? *Do your research. Ask questions.* My intent is not to "bust" my colleagues but to help you have a smile that reveals who you really are!

I consider this to be *the* most important chapter of all, and here's why: Simply showing different methods of improving your smile means nothing if you choose the wrong dentist to perform your procedure. Every person wants different kinds of services from his or her dentist; it's up you to choose the one that fits you best. So be sure to do your research well!

＊

Chapter 9
Caring for Your Beautiful Smile

We all know we should brush at least twice a day, floss once a day, and see the dentist every six months or so, yet most people don't follow these simple suggestions. Still, prevention and maintenance are the best ways to care for your smile. So follow this advice if you want to know that you are doing everything you can to take the best care of your mouth at home. The selection of products and tools you purchase to care for your smile *does* matter.

The overall goal of home care is to remove plaque (dental biofilm) and bacteria. Retaining plaque leads to cavities and gum disease, and it ultimately can shorten the lifespan of any cosmetic dentistry in your mouth. The sticky film of bacteria needs to be removed via brushing and flossing, or it can cause anything from enamel breakdown to gum disease. After you eat, the bacteria release acids that attack tooth enamel. Most of the 600 species of bacteria that may be found in the mouth are likely to be harmless, but some are known to be involved in oral disease.

If you eat sugary foods without cleaning well afterward, plaque thrives on that sugar. As soon as it accumulates, acids will start to break down the enamel, demineralizing its protective coating and encouraging cavities to form. As noted earlier, when plaque stays on the teeth long enough, it hardens and eventually turns into tartar, also called "calculus." This is what your hygienist scrapes off at your cleaning appointments.

The presence of plaque on gums and tooth surfaces can also cause inflammation of the gums, commonly referred to as "gingivitis." Gums become red, swollen, and irritated, and they tend to bleed easily. The plaque can easily creep down below the gum line, causing bone loss and eventual tooth loss. If gingivitis goes untreated, inflammation spreads to the gums around the base of the tooth and causes a condition called "periodontitis." Eventually, this disease can erode the bone around the tooth, causing tooth loss.

One recent review suggests that 50 percent of all age groups in the U.S. population have reversible gingival inflammation, with moderate to severe periodontitis affecting 5 to 15 percent of the population.[2]

Needless to say, if you take care of your teeth and gums, you greatly reduce the chance of losing your teeth. Aging doesn't necessarily correlate to tooth loss; tooth loss is preventable. The teeth and gums need to be cleaned through brushing and

---

2 G.W. Taylor and W.S. Borgnakke, "Periodontal disease: associations with diabetes, glycemic control and complications," *Oral Diseases* 14 (2008): 191-203.

flossing, while adjunct methods such as rinsing with mouth-wash and tongue scraping certainly help. A number of newly published studies in the *Journal of Periodontology* confirm recent findings that people with periodontal disease are at a greater risk of systemic diseases, such as cardiovascular disease.

Here's how that happens: Researchers have found that diseased gums release higher levels of bacterial pro-inflam-matory components into the bloodstream. These components can find their way to other organs, including the heart, and increase their risk of failure. In fact, studies have shown that heart disease may actually originate in the mouth. Specifi-cally, the September 2009 issue of *Cancer Epidemiology, Biomark-ers, and Prevention* states, "The health hazards associated with chronic periodontitis (gum disease) extend way beyond the mouth. For years people have been warned that persistent periodontitis can cause heart disease. Now a new study sug-gests that gum disease may also be a risk factor for cancers of the head and neck."[3]

The link between oral and systemic health is strengthened every day through new and ongoing research. The possibility of preventing heart attack, stroke, diabetes, pulmonary and kidney diseases, Alzheimer's disease, pregnancy complications, and cancers of many kinds should give you plenty of incentive to practice excellent oral hygiene!

Toothbrushes: Many times while shopping, I've watched a person pause for what seems an eternity in front of the aisle containing the vast number of choices for toothbrushes, tooth-pastes, mouthwashes, and floss. What's best? Consider tooth-brushes. The ideal toothbrush should safely remove plaque as

---

3 Mine Tezal et al., "Chronic Periodontitis and the Incidence of Head and Neck Squamous Cell Carcinoma," *Cancer Epidemiology, Biomarkers & Prevention* 18 (September 2009): 2406-2412.

efficiently as possible as it delivers the toothpaste to the tooth surface without damaging the teeth or gums. It should be easy to use and should remove the plaque from the whole tooth surface—even between the teeth.

Toothbrushes are generally sold in three bristle stiffness levels—soft, medium, and hard. We recommend using soft bristles because hard and even medium can damage your gums. Also, an electric toothbrush can help you brush your teeth

Here's How to Brush Properly

- No matter what toothbrush you select, speak to your dentist or hygienist about the proper way to use it! As long as you're brushing correctly, any brush will do the trick.
- It's important to brush all the surfaces of your teeth—cheek side, tongue side, and chewing surface.
- Hold the brush at a 45-degree angle to the tooth so the bristles face up toward the gums. Press firmly so the bristles reach into the spaces between your gums and teeth.
- Don't brush hard or aggressively; brush only as hard as it takes to get between your teeth. Certainly don't take out your day's frustrations on your teeth. Brushing too hard can actually wear your enamel and dentin away, as well as cause your gums to recede. Instead, use short, circular motions, spending about 10 seconds in each area you're cleaning.
- Even though twice a day is a general rule, it's helpful to brush after meals, so even three to four times daily isn't overdoing it. If you can't brush after a meal, take a moment to rinse with water or chew sugar-free gum.

Remember, *how* you brush is just as important as *when* or *how often* you brush. Ask your hygienist to show you any areas of your mouth you're missing when you brush and how to clean them better.

more effectively. You simply hold the moving brush against your teeth for at least two minutes and let it do all the work for you.

Experiment by using a manual, a powered, and a sonic brush. Powered brushes have been found to remove more plaque in the same amount of time as a manual brush. Ultrasonic toothbrushes can give you a "professional," clean feeling and are available from your dentist or drugstore for $90 to $150. Different ones boast different features, so ask your dentist which is best for you. New ultrasonics feature timers so you'll brush for an adequate amount of time, about two minutes. (Yes, two whole minutes! One study noted that the average American brushes for 39 seconds, not two minutes!)

A rule of thumb is to replace your toothbrush every two to three months, or even sooner if the bristles get frayed or flattened. Remember, toothbrushes can house a lot of bacteria, including E. coli, so rinse your brush thoroughly and let it air dry. Never share your brush with someone else, because you risk transmitting decay and gum disease. Likewise, throw your brush away after you've been sick with a cold or infection.

Seeing your dentist for regular cleanings and checkups helps prevent big problems by catching and addressing small ones. When you visit, maintaining your cosmetic work may take a few extra steps, but it will be well worth the extra effort to help your new smile last longer.

You may want to ask your dentist for a recommendation regarding toothpaste, floss, and mouth rinses because various kinds claim to do various things. Or do your own research by reading the packaging carefully before you buy. Again, *what* you use is less important than *how* you use it.

Toothpastes: You have so many options for toothpastes that choosing one can become overwhelming. I'll attempt to help you sort it out.

A number of ingredients are necessary to help toothpaste taste, feel, and perform the way it should. Fluoride is the one essential ingredient because it helps prevent decay and improves gum health by decreasing the ability of bacteria to stick to the tooth surface. It also improves a tooth's overall hardness. In fact, the ADA agrees that fluoride has been proven to decrease decay by 60 percent.

Toothpastes claim many benefits, such as whitening, fresh breath, plaque and gingivitis removal, tartar control, and desensitizing. While most toothpastes contain ingredients to provide all these benefits, most of them target one problem

What Toothpaste Do You Use on Veneers?

The number one question asked after our clients get veneers is this: "What toothpaste do I use?" While some toothpastes are better than others for use on porcelain veneers, no product specifically for veneers has existed—until now.

Smile Stylist has formulated a dual-power porcelain-polishing toothpaste designed for people who have cosmetic dentistry. The reality is that more and more people have cosmetic porcelain crowns, veneers, and white fillings, and toothpaste has not changed to better protect the new components of people's teeth and smiles. Smile Stylist porcelain-polishing toothpaste combines ingredients used in our office to polish porcelain and bondings with ingredients used in home-care toothpastes to keep the teeth clean and polished. The Smile Stylist low-abrasivity formulation is gentle on cosmetic dental work and employs the newest technology and ingredients to fight cavities and strengthen teeth.

and address it. Again, the most important ingredient is fluoride. Once it's incorporated into the tooth structure, it strengthens the tooth, making it more resistant to cavities.

This may surprise you, but whitening toothpastes do *not* whiten teeth. Brushing with toothpaste may remove superficial stains caused by coffee, for instance, and thus make the teeth *appear* lighter, but the actual tooth is not lighter. Be careful. Some whitening toothpastes may be too abrasive and damage your enamel over a number of years.

Toothpastes are measured by their RDA (relative dentin abrasivity). You don't want your toothpaste to be highly abrasive, because using abrasive toothpastes may actually wear down or sand down your tooth enamel. Ask your dentist which toothpastes may be too abrasive for you. We recommend a toothpaste with a low RDA rating, especially if your teeth are sensitive, which is a common problem. Sixty percent of Americans have sensitivity issues with their teeth. Their teeth can be sensitive to cold and heat, sweets, or brushing. Desensitizing toothpastes use potassium nitrate, sodium citrate, or strontium to block the nerve channels by sealing up the dentin tubules that guard the nerves, thus preventing sensitivity. I recommend a toothpaste called Sensodyne for people who have sensitive teeth.

Flossing: A common saying among dentists is "Floss only the teeth you want to keep." I'm sure many dentists share this with their patients as well. It seems people hate flossing, but it's essential to oral health. Why? Because flossing removes plaque and trapped food from between the teeth and below the gum line, and it stimulates the gums. A toothbrush simply can't reach between the teeth or where the teeth contact each other, yet commonly cavities start there. Stimulating the gums keeps them healthy and tight.

Many patients ask why their gums bleed when they floss only once in a while. This may be normal for anyone who doesn't floss regularly. Bleeding should decrease and even disappear with regular flossing. Even people who floss often may not be doing it correctly. Dentists recommend the technique of wrapping the floss around your tooth and moving it up and down, not sawing it back and forth. On your next visit, your hygienist can show you how to floss effectively. Also, a number of aids are available to help facilitate flossing.

Bad Breath: Once you have a gorgeous smile, you'll want to show it off to everyone you're with, so don't let bad breath stand in your way. Most people have bad breath in the morning or after eating onions and garlic (transitory bad breath), but about 80 million people have halitosis (chronic bad breath), a condition that's considerably worse than morning breath. It's from bacteria in the mouth that cause gases to be released. The bacteria come from food particles that get stuck in hard-to-reach places such as between the teeth, under the gums, or on the back of the tongue. These food particles attract bacteria that form colonies and ferment. This in turn produces volatile sulphur compounds that have an unpleasant smell.

Add 6.4 Years to Your Life—Floss!

On **November 14, 2009**, *Early Show Saturday Edition* on the CBS television network featured a program called "Quick Fixes to Add Years to Your Life!" about things we can control to live longer. The researchers on the program noted that *flossing* can add an extra 6.4 years of life because it helps control periodontal disease and reduces the chance of bacteria invading the fatty substances in arteries, which can lead to strokes and heart attacks. Another excellent reason to floss.

Do This Bad Breath Self-Test

How do you know if you have bad breath? It's hard to detect it on yourself, and most people won't tell their loved ones, friends, or colleagues that they find their breath offensive. However, you can do this self-test: Lick the back of your hand, wait 5 to 10 seconds, then smell it. If it smells bad to you, chances are it smells bad to everyone around you as well.

The majority of bad breath originates from the tongue—an area people commonly forget to clean. Your tongue has fibers that are loaded with bacteria, particularly at the back of the tongue. Brushing—or even better, scraping—your tongue should be added to your home care regimen. In most cases, proper home care can decrease bad breath. We don't recommend masking bad breath with mouthwashes, mints, or gum. Most mouthwashes work only for about 10 minutes or so anyway.

Other causes of bad breath include dry mouth, some medicines, dieting, smoking, and alcohol. Ways to fight bad breath include

- home care (brushing, flossing, tongue scraping);
- watching your diet (avoiding garlic and onions, which produce gases that cause bad breath, and eating more fruits and veggies);
- drinking plenty of water; and
- chewing sugarless gum to create more saliva (thus eliminating dry mouth, one cause of bad breath).

Now you know the many ways a smile can be enhanced and how to take good care of your smile. Check out our website, www.smilestylist.com, to see many more incredible smile makeovers. You can read about how these improvements have changed lives.

My husband and I drive to work every day feeling so excited about the patients we're going to see. We feel so lucky! We have the best jobs in the world. People often don't realize how much an embarrassing smile can affect their life. Once they receive their new smile, it's amazing to see these people act on the outside how they've always felt on the inside. Their self-confidence soars, and we love helping them celebrate by photographing their happy new look. Check out their new smiles!

Meet the Smile Stylists, Dr. Colleen Olitsky and Dr. Jason Olitsky

I, Colleen, am part of the team at the Smile Stylists, the dental studio I share with my husband, Jason Olitsky, DMD, an experienced cosmetic dentist. I am also the author of *Style Your Smile*, a book that contains dozens of photographs I use to help clients understand their treatment options.

Both Jason and I graduated from Temple University's School of Dentistry in 2001. While there, we received very little training in cosmetic dentistry. However, when we learned the incredible value of this special field, we began our quest to become leaders in it. We both feel that smiles are vastly underrepresented in the media given the importance Americans place on them in our culture. Many surveys have highlighted this fact. By working with publicists, writing books, developing products, and managing models with beautiful smiles, we hope to get more representation of smiles in national media—similar to the attention given to hair, skin, makeup, and clothing. Why?

Because currently only about 20 percent of the U.S. population goes to the dentist regularly, and many systemic life-threatening illnesses are exacerbated by poor oral health. If we can raise awareness among the population to take better care of their oral health, we can have a direct impact on the seriousness of those illnesses.

In the last eight years, both of us have taken more than a thousand hours of continuing education, learning from the top cosmetic dentistry instructors in the country. It has paid off. Jason now teaches with his mentor, David Hornbrook, DDS, FAACD, initially for the Hornbrook Group, and now for Gold Dust Clinical Mastery. When he was recruiting faculty for his center, Dr. Hornbrook found just twenty people who met his strict criteria. Jason is also an adjunct faculty member of the Arizona School of Dentistry & Oral Health.

I've assisted Jason on every case at our office. We uphold the highest standards in cosmetic dentistry, and it shows. For example, our client Whitney Thompson was the winner of Cycle 10 of *America's Next Top Model*, and the smile makeover we performed on her was featured on the cover of the 2009 summer edition of *The Journal of Cosmetic Dentistry*, the official publication of the seven-thousand-member American Academy of Cosmetic Dentistry (AACD).

Both Jason and I have given presentations at dental conventions, including the AACD, the Florida Academy of Cosmetic Dentistry (Jason serves on its board), and the Academy of Comprehensive Esthetics. Topics include marketing, branding, trademarks, and smile design.

As a member of the AACD, Jason is working toward accreditation in cosmetic dentistry. As of this writing, only 250 dentists in the entire world have become accredited. He has passed all five accreditation cases thus far, and Jason has simply to pass the oral exam in order to join that elite group of dentists.

Jason and I have been quoted as experts on cosmetic

dentistry in *Self*, *Fitness*, *Real Simple*, *Women's Health*, and *First Magazine*. Our success has been highlighted in Blatchford Blueprints, written by Dr. Bill and Carolyn Blatchford, as well as in an article in the April 2006 issue of *Dental Economics*. In addition, we've been interviewed eight times, collectively, on all three TV news stations in Jacksonville, Florida.

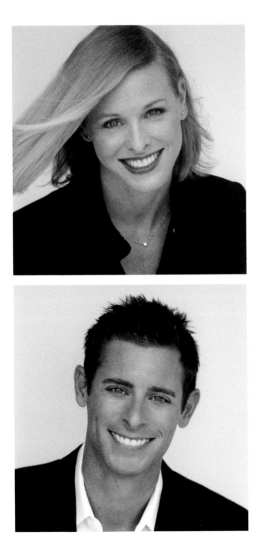

❋

Acknowledgments

What a fun journey thus far! There are many people to thank, but I will keep it brief.

Jason, thanks for all of your love, patience, and support, both emotional and technical.

Dr. David Hornbrook, thanks for inspiring us to be the best we can be.

Gold Dust Dental Lab, thanks for providing us with such stunning ceramics.

Dr. Bill and Carolyn Blatchford, thanks for helping us dream big.

Jamie Lynch, thanks for all of your belief, passion, and energy in Smile Stylist.

Lisa Kaminski, thanks for all you do for our studio.

Our parents, you guys are the best, we love you!!!

Baby Chase, you definitely made this adventure much harder and we love you for it, thanks for not being boring!